I0408052

Fibromyalgia For Life:

Living Well With A Difficult Disease

Kara Owl

The scanning, uploading and distribution of this book via the Internet or via any other means without the permission of the publisher is illegal and punishable by law. Please purchase only authorized editions and do not participate in or encourage the electronic piracy of copyrighted materials. Your support of the author's rights is appreciated.

This is a work of nonfiction. Names used within this work are either used with the permission of the individual, or are names used to protect the identity of those who chose not to reveal their names. No warranty is implied or given about the use of tarot. This book is not intended to treat or diagnose any medical condition.

FIBROMYALGIA FOR LIFE: LIVING WELL WITH A DIFFICULT DISEASE
ALL RIGHTS RESERVED
Copyright © Kara Owl, 2013
Cover Art ® 2013 by Winterheart Design
Edited by Mary K. Wilson
ISBN# 978-1542734240
Electronic Publication Date: January 2017
Print Publication Date: January 2017

This book may not be reproduced or used in whole or in part by any means existing without written permission from the publisher.

For more information to learn to more about this, or any other Kara Owl publication, please visit
www.facebook.com/WriterKaraOwl/

Contents

Introduction

In 1997 I was diagnosed with fibromyalgia. I did as much research as I could, but the information I could get my hands on at the time was sparse and often contradictory. Doctors told me not to do things that hurt, which for me included exercise. They prescribed me medications that made me fat, dizzy, and unable to think. After years of struggling I finally found a doctor who listened to me, and I was able to go off all the medications as she encouraged me to listen to my body and try various holistic treatments. With a change of diet, exercise, and pain management, I finally managed to control the fibro, as much as I can. I don't want anyone to go through what I went through, and that is what pushed the creation of this book.

We are all individuals, and fibro will hurt in different ways for different people. One thing is certain: we all need to learn how to treat our pain in the way which works best for us. For some, diet changes may help, especially if your fibro pain is exacerbated by IBS (Irritable Bowel Syndrome) or a food allergy. Fibromyalgia often doesn't occur alone; it comes with friends, which makes treatment and diagnosis interesting at times. Other individuals may need exercise programs, to help the muscles to stretch and stay flexible. For a few, pain medication may be the only way to treat it. Trial and error will lead us to our way, and once we find it we can live a happy and full life despite the fibro.

This book is not a "guide to fixing fibro," nor is it a "one true way" treatise. Rather, the one thing I have learned from my decade-plus battle with fibro is that there is no one true way for everyone. I will relate things that other sufferers have told me, cite research that has been done to find helpful practices, and talk of the things that have worked for me, but you will have to find your own path through this wild illness.

One thing I will say: there is a lot of hard, medical evidence that fibro is real. Don't let anyone tell you it's not. There are a lot of male sufferers out there, too, so don't let anyone tell you it's a "woman's disease." While researching this book I met a great deal of men with fibro who asked me to make sure that I included them, because they felt invisible both to the fibro community and to some doctors, who were convinced they couldn't have fibro because they were men. A study done in the 1990s bears out that while the majority of sufferers are women, nearly 14% of those with fibro are men.

This book is for everyone. I even include a few words here and there for the spouses and partners of fibro sufferers, because they are going through this with us as well. Together, we can all find our way to overcome the obstacles this illness puts in front of us.

We may have fibromyalgia, but it doesn't have us!

Chapter 1—What is Fibromyalgia?

Fibromyalgia is a poorly understood illness. Sadly, even some doctors don't accept that it is a real illness. And so, when you or someone you love receives a diagnosis of fibromyalgia, you're facing a wall of misinformation, myth, and rumors that have a lot of people thinking people with fibro are weak, lazy, or hypochondriacs.

Fibromyalgia is a real medical condition. It is not a psychiatric condition. It is not "just in your head." It is not just you being "sensitive" or having a "low pain tolerance." It's real and it's treatable. If you suspect you or someone you love has it, you should first see a doctor for a diagnosis. While there are medications and treatment plans that can help make it more bearable, the first step is always confirmation with a medical professional. There are many illnesses that mimic the symptoms of fibromyalgia, so you must first rule out other problems, some of which are more serious. Once you have the diagnosis of fibromyalgia, you may then move on to finding treatments that work for you.

What fibromyalgia is exactly and what causes it are not completely understood yet. The symptoms, however, are clear: they are widespread musculoskeletal pain, fatigue, a lack of restful or restorative sleep, and at least 11 of 18 specific tender points radiating pain when pressed.

In order for fibromyalgia to be diagnosed, you must experience the pain and fatigue for at least three months, and doctors must rule out other similar illnesses such as Lupus or depression, which also cause pain and fatigue.

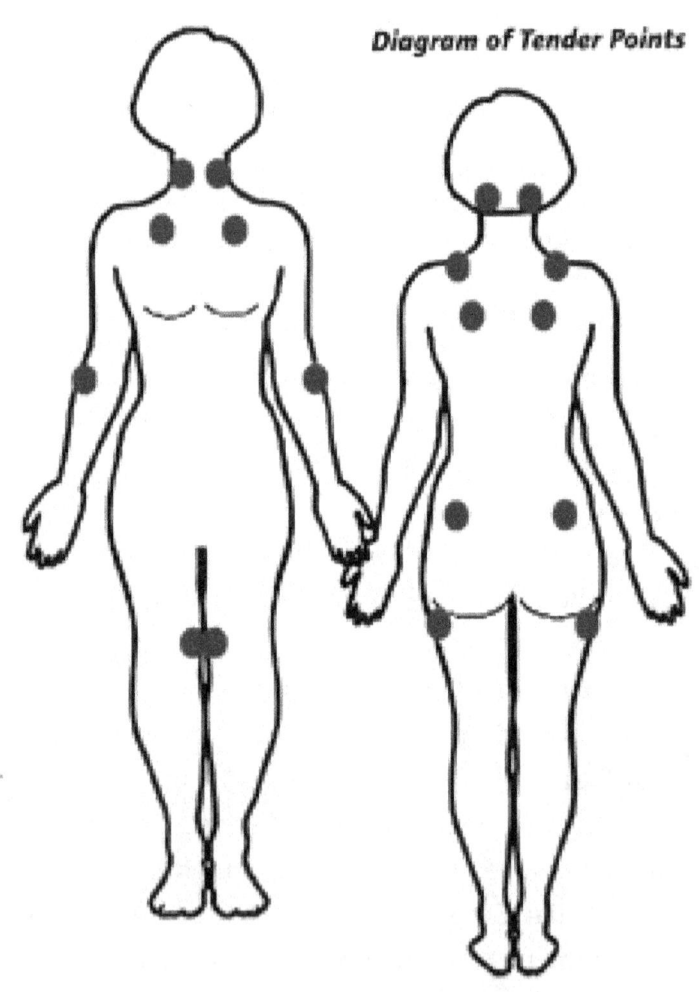

Diagram of Tender Points

There are many treatments for fibro, including physical therapy, cognitive-behavioral therapy, and various medications, including fibro-specific medications like Lyrica or Savella. It is important to see a doctor to determine if these treatments will work for you and to rule out more severe illnesses.

Lupus is debilitating, painful, and can be fatal if it goes untreated. Fibro is difficult to live with, but it will not kill you. It may make you wish you were dead, particularly if you're dealing with other people who don't understand it, but the one small blessing is that it is not usually degenerative.

The biggest issue with fibro is the lack of restful, restorative sleep. In sleep studies done on people with fibro, the researchers observed that fibro patients never achieved deep sleep (slow wave sleep), often woke frequently through the night, had difficulty falling asleep, and never achieved the kind of restful sleep that is needed to repair the body and refresh the mind.

Of course, this is a "chicken and egg" scenario. Which came first, the lack of restful sleep, or the fibromyalgia? So far, researchers have not clearly identified the cause of fibro, but it is being actively investigated. Hopefully, they'll find a cause that will lead them to a cure.

In addition to the basic issues that fibro creates, it is often accompanied by sensitivity to foods, smells, and allergens, gastrointestinal issues, and psychiatric issues such as depression. All of these must be treated in order for the fibro sufferer to regain his or her former life. This is also why it is imperative that you see a doctor for an initial diagnosis, so that you can put together a medical team that helps you to find your way back to good (or at least better) health. There is still a stigma associated with fibromyalgia, and it can be difficult to find a good doctor for treatment, but they are out there. Keep searching, don't give up, and don't let the fibro get you down.

Chapter 2—The Science and the Myth

Fibromyalgia is a confusing disease, especially since there has been a lot of misinformation out there. In this chapter, I'm going to discuss what it is, what it isn't, debunk common myths, and hopefully help you understand fibromyalgia a bit better.

Fibromyalgia has undergone a lot of change since the doctors 'discovered' it a few decades ago. Initially, it was thought to be an autoimmune disorder similar to Lupus. Research debunked that, so then they thought it was similar to arthritis. However, in arthritic joints and muscles, there is a great deal of inflammation and damage. In fibro, these things do not occur—there's no visible sign of fibro, other than the tender points and cluster of symptoms.

Currently, doctors believe that fibro is its own disease, with a specific cluster of symptoms. However, they also have discovered that each individual with fibro reacts to their symptoms in a body-specific manner. And so treatment is hit-and-miss as each person and his or her doctor uncover a path to a happier, healthier life with fibro.

In a 1990 study by Dr. Carol Jessup, she found that nearly 100% of people with fibro had specific issues including chronic fatigue, memory impairment, and cold extremities. Nearly 90% of her subjects had yeast overgrowth. She speculated that the imbalance may have led to the other symptoms and thus the fibro.

People with fibro have a higher than normal incidence of PTSD. This has led some researchers to speculate that trauma may lead to sensitivities to "substance P," which is a pain receptor. The sensitivity to this pain receptor then could lead to the individual feeling greater pain than usual, and the pain creates a cascade that leads to the other symptoms of fibro. This is not proven, other than the fact that people with fibro do have a greater amount of, or sensitivity to, substance P.

Currently, doctors attempt to treat fibro by treating the symptoms. This can be frustrating for the person with fibro, because the symptoms are so varied. People with fibro may end up seeing a psychiatrist for their depression, a general practitioner for their pain, and a gastroenterologist for the bowel issues that often accompany fibro, among myriad other doctors! We have to be careful to manage our doctors, keeping everyone in the loop of what treatments are ongoing, and that can be troublesome thanks to the memory issues we all suffer with.

Until the research community comes through with a more focused cause that we can treat, however, all we can do is manage our symptoms.

The biggest symptom and issue in fibromyalgia is the interrupted sleep, which is not restful and does not allow the body to repair itself the way that normal sleep does. And so, current research clusters around figuring out which came first—the lack of restful sleep, or the fibro? As of this writing, several articles in Science Daily and at WebMD discuss sleep habits and fibro, and it seems that a great deal of research is being sent towards finding out what will help with this issue.

As mentioned earlier, research has also proven that people with fibro have higher than normal levels of "substance P," a neurotransmitter associated with pain. Blood tests on people with fibromyalgia show substance P at levels three times higher than "normal" people. And so, research is trying to determine why, how these levels originate, and thus uncover the root cause of fibromyalgia. Hopefully, these developments will lead to a better treatment, or even perhaps to a cure.

Sadly, all this science still has not removed several myths from surrounding fibromyalgia and creating a lot of frustration for people who have the illness. Including the ever-popular "it's all in your head."

Fibromyalgia is not just in the sufferer's head. As stated above, there is proof now that fibromyalgia is not imaginary, is not psychiatric, and definitely causes physical pain and suffering for each individual who has it. Aside from the higher levels of substance P, fibro sufferers also have a specific pattern of poor sleep that can be seen during a sleep study.

Sadly, even some doctors still hold to the "it's a myth" attitude, and thus cause more issues for people with fibro. It is imperative that if you are told this by a doctor, you fire that doctor and find another. It is NOT in your head. On the plus side, thanks to the research that is being undertaken by reputable colleges and doctors, that attitude is diminishing.

The subset of that myth that is exceedingly irksome is that fibro patients "fake" their pain, or simply have a low pain tolerance. Nothing could be farther from the truth. The neurotransmitters are out of whack in our bodies, and so we experience pain differently. That does not mean that we are 'faking' or that we have a low pain tolerance. I know fibro patients who say that broken bones or kidney stones are not as bad as their fibro pain. While I'm not in that boat (my experience with a kidney stone was horrid!), I believe them. Pain is relative—we are not wimps; we simply deal with more pain on a regular basis than most people do.

Another myth is that this is a "woman's disease." Fibromyalgia can strike anyone. Children, men, the elderly, and yes—women. As mentioned earlier, the current ratio seems to be 14% men to 86% women according to a 2002 study published in the Journal of American Medicine. There's a subset of this myth that I recently came across, a belief that it only hits white people. In actuality, in a study at the University of California-San Francisco shows that fibromyalgia is actually more common among African-Americans, though the ratio was very close. (This study was published in the Journal of Rheumatology in 2007.) The sub-myth here is that you are "too young" for fibro, or at the other extreme, that it's "just old age." Fibro can strike anyone, young and old. Younger people with fibro have a horrible time being diagnosed, because they are dismissed as being too young for this kind of pain. My advice to them and their parents is to persist, because it's real and it does hit children. On the other end, people being dismissed as "just getting older" also need to keep fighting. It's not necessarily "just old age." Fibro pain is something different, and if you think you've got it, find a good doctor or keep searching until you get the answers you need and deserve.

A third common myth involves exercise. Some say people with fibro should never exercise, while others say exercise will fix everything! In actuality, fibromyalgia is very body-specific, and so individuals must learn their own limits, and uncover what helps and hurts on their own. In general, yoga and gentle stretching do help, and will also improve your mood if you add upbeat meditations to the end of your yoga routine. (I use Rodney Yee's yoga routines, which include a calming mediation at the end, and they are very helpful to me.) However, exercise will not magically fix everything! And those who perpetuate this myth need to understand that fibro is a real condition with real issues. A subset of this myth is that fibro sufferers "just need to push through the pain."

NO! This is a dangerous idea, even for healthy people! Pain generally means there is a problem. This can be problematic for fibro sufferers who are constantly in pain. We speak, here, of sudden and sharp pains, or of pain levels higher than those with which you generally deal. If you feel this kind of pain while exercising, you need to stop doing what you're doing. NEVER "push through" *pain*. Discomfort, yes, you can attempt to push through or stretch to relieve it. You can "push through" your usual pain levels in order to be able to exercise. But if you feel a sudden, sharp pain, stop! If your pain levels suddenly rise while exercising, stop! The idea that anyone would tell even a healthy person to push through pain is incredibly infuriating to me—that people say this to people with fibro makes me so enraged I want to find these people and inflict fibro on them! This is absolutely a myth, and one that I'm happy to debunk.

Corollary to the exercise myth are a large number of food and drink myths. People with fibro mustn't eat certain foods, or drink certain drinks, or take caffeine in any way, or eat white sugar, etc. Again, this goes back to the fact that fibro is body specific. A large number of people with fibro are gluten intolerant. But *not all!* And so, for some people cutting out gluten will help immensely. For others, there will be no difference. The same goes for caffeine, sugar, and any other food people can get up in arms about. For some fibro sufferers, it'll be a godsend to avoid that. For others, they'll be cranky and tired in addition to their usual pain.

The flipside of this myth is the "take [insert vitamin here/colloidal silver/guiafenesin/etc] and you'll be cured!" I have heard so many people say that various drugs, vitamins, and substances "fixed" their fibro. Vitamin D and the various B-vitamins (particularly B6 and B12) seem to be the most common "cures." Again, if they work for you, fantastic! Take your vitamins and enjoy your improved health. But the supplements won't work for 100% of fibro patients, so please don't go around saying that you've "found the cure." It's a cure for you, and that's great, but it probably won't fix all the people you meet with fibro. And beware any site that says "we cure fibro!" They're definitely selling something.

Along the same lines, I've heard so many times "if you just lose weight, you'll feel better!" Some of my skinny fibro-friends hear the opposite: "just gain some weight, you'll feel better!" That's false, and it's been debunked by many people who have lost (or gained) weight and still hurt. When I first got fibro, I was in amazing shape, working out multiple days a week, hiking and horseback riding, and staying very active. I didn't start hearing the "lose weight, you'll feel better" until I had gained about 40 lbs. The first time I heard it, I told a doctor "I got this illness when I was thin." He didn't believe me. The knots in our muscles don't care how much weight we bear. They are going to hurt, despite weight loss or gain.

The knots in a fibro sufferer's muscles are groups of muscle fibers that tighten over time, and don't release the way that muscles are designed to release. The knots are generally found near tender points, the spots that a doctor presses on to find out if you have fibro. They will feel like small bumps or nodules if you are able to find them while doing a self-massage. These are the source of a great deal of the pain that we must cope with.

People with fibro also get informed that they'll never have a 'normal' relationship, or worse—told they shouldn't have sex. I will discuss sex in more detail later, but I'd like to reassure any fibro sufferers whose well-meaning friends have said they shouldn't have sex that people with fibro are like any other person with a chronic pain condition or disability. There are going to be times where they won't be able to or want to have sex because of their pain. That doesn't mean they can't or shouldn't.

They should do what they want to do, when they want, and have the energy to do it.

As to the normal relationship, is any relationship normal? I don't think so. And I think—speaking as a woman who's been married for over a decade now—that people with fibro can have happy, healthy, successful relationships if they want. And they can also be happy living the single life, too, if that's what they choose! The fibro is a problem, but you don't need to avoid relationships or sex because of it. You may need to search harder for a partner who will accept you despite your limitations, but they are out there. Keep searching until you find the right person for you.

I have heard a lot of mixed information about what fibro is and isn't. As of this writing, fibro is not classified as an autoimmune disease or a form of arthritis. It doesn't cause the inflammation associated with these illnesses. I've also heard that fibro causes Lupus, or that it's fatal. Fibro definitely doesn't *cause* Lupus, though it can be concurrent with Lupus, and I know many people who bear both illnesses. Fibro is also not fatal. In rare cases, it can be degenerative, but it is not a fatal illness.

Of course, the biggest issue facing people with fibro is that our disease is invisible. The "but you look fine!" exclamation is frustrating and sometimes belittling. As though we have no right to be sick, because we look fine. I try to deal gracefully with this, but it is not always easy. My standard reply is "thank you, it's good to know I don't look as bad as I feel." And, it's good to have a standard response for this particular annoying statement, because you'll likely hear it a lot.

Worse than that, though, is when people say "oh, just don't think about the pain." This particular comment is another infuriating one. It's demeaning, and it implies that our pain is just in our heads and we should somehow magically be able to ignore it. I say "would you tell someone with the flu to ignore their pain?" and attempt to force them to realize that the pain is not imaginary or ignorable. It doesn't always work, but the times it does make the effort worth it.

I am sure there are more fibro myths that I have forgotten or left out. There is so much misinformation out there about this illness. It's incredibly frustrating, and there is only so much energy that we have for correcting it. Hopefully, as word gets out, the misinformation will vanish as more people are educated about our illness.

Until then, we will do our best!

Chapter 3—After the Diagnosis, now what?

You've been in horrible pain for ages and finally your doctor gives you a diagnosis: "it's fibromyalgia." What does that mean? What do you do now?

Well, the dry, science-filled answer is that fibromyalgia is a chronic pain disorder characterized by widespread musculoskeletal pain, fatigue, and tender points. It is treatable, but as yet incurable. Those are the facts, but what do they really mean for you?

It means that your muscles hurt. Your joints hurt. You're tired no matter how much you sleep. Your body is tender, and sometimes even wearing clothes hurts or bothers you. It means that at specific points on your body, you have extra pain and muscle knots. The tender points make other areas hurt and exacerbate sleep issues. It means that you have an excessive sensitivity to chemical smells. You may even find sounds that you can't handle, and that produce a physical reaction. It means you may have skin allergies or irritations. All this and more I haven't mentioned might be part of what fibromyalgia does to you.

While you probably want to start treatment immediately, what need to do is give yourself space and time to absorb the diagnosis and grieve for your old life. It's not easy to adjust to a chronic, incurable illness. Even when you know you can treat it, even when you have a plan, you're still going to resent the changes you need to make in your lifestyle, feel envious of your friends who don't have to deal with this, and need time and space to adjust to your new limitations. This is a process, and it may take a while. I have had this illness for a long time, and I still have moments where I have to pause and grieve what I've lost, or rage against the injustice. And there are still times where I have to reassess my treatment plan, to make it work the best for me.

While it may seem cliché, people with fibro do go through the five stages of grief. We may go through them differently. We may get stuck in one. We may go from denial to grief to anger and back to denial again, but grief is a process, and every person with a chronic illness gets to go through it.

After you are diagnosed, you will likely find yourself in denial. Even if you accept the fibro diagnosis, you may find yourself thinking, saying, or hoping "it won't really last forever, right?" You may try to continue your old life. You may find yourself pushing, until you crash and burn and the fibro flares until you can't ignore it.

It's normal. Don't beat yourself up for doing this. Don't beat yourself up for doing this a few times as you learn your limitations. It takes time, patience, and experience to accept your new normal, and you're going to have to overdo it a few times before you figure out what is 'too much' activity, or too many people, or even learn what triggers your particular sensitivities.

One 'stage' that I have mentally added to the stages of grief for people with chronic illnesses is the "research" stage. It doesn't fit in any of the current stages, though I suppose it could be a type of bargaining ("If I learn everything about this, I will be able to beat it!"). It is, quite literally, a quest. A quest for something that will fix the illness.

In this stage, the person afflicted hunts out and often tries every crazy and realistic method to cure what ails them—in this case, fibro. Often, a doctor will help them, since some doctors don't believe in fibro. If a particular doctor won't help them, though, they'll hunt out a new one who will. They research the illness; they read books; they try medications and meditations and everything in between.

It is a part of the process, and if you're recognizing yourself in it, don't fret. I did it, too.

For me, the process was denial, bargaining, denial, research, denial, depression, acceptance. Though, some people would say that I haven't quite achieved acceptance, since I still occasionally struggle with pushing too far or with anger at my limitations. I think these people have too high of an expectation for what "acceptance" really is. I believe it's a process. Yes, certainly, sometimes you'll slide back into anger or bargaining or depression—but I think total acceptance of something like fibro involves the occasional flash of anger at the limitations, or swoop of sadness at what you've lost.

I don't think a bit of anger or sadness constitute a lack of acceptance. I think they're normal human emotions that are going to happen from time to time.

This is a new you, and the old you has to find out how this crazy new you fits, and some bits will chafe, and some bits will be too big, and there's no real way to tailor this new you to fit as well as the old one may have. It will take time to adjust, and you will need to be patient while you settle in to the new you.

Once you have adjusted to your new reality, then you must learn your new limitations, what will exhaust you, what will energize you, what hurts and what doesn't. For some people with fibro, those limitations will be severe. Everything hurts, and so they will need to adjust schedules, limit their activities, and perhaps give up beloved jobs or hobbies. For others, their limitations will not be as problematic, and they'll be able to resume their ordinary life after adding medications or beginning a gentle stretching or yoga routine.

You may find that you need more time doing your usual activities. When I was diagnosed, I discovered everything takes longer. I used to be able to shower in the morning in five to ten minutes, hop out of the shower and get dressed, and be out of the house in 30 minutes. Now, I find that showering takes longer, and sometimes I have to take a moment once I'm out of the shower to stretch muscles that haven't loosened up as much as I thought they would, or to rest because even though the hot shower helped the pain, it also sapped some of my precious energy.

I also recommend you gently push your limits. Be cautious, but try and do as much as you can to keep yourself active. Despite the conventional wisdom when I was first diagnosed, staying flexible—in body and mind—seems to help a great deal with controlling fibromyalgia pain. I found the more I exercised, the better I felt. Most people with fibro find that a gentle yoga routine greatly helps with their mental clarity and physical pain levels. For some, even more than that will be good. I have a friend with fibro who lifts weights, another is exploring ice skating, and a third runs. Studies have shown that aerobic exercise helps a great deal. Water aerobics is apparently the most helpful thing, but it can be difficult to find a swimming pool that is close enough to your house to get to without a lot of trouble. Still, try things to see what works for you, and don't let the naysayers stop you.

There will always be people who will worry, who will say "you shouldn't do that" because of the fibro. Don't listen to them; listen to your body. If your body is saying that it helps, keep it up. Well-meaning people can sometimes be your worst enemies. They will try to wrap you in bubble wrap and keep you "safe," but for us there is no such thing. We need to find our own best path, and for those of us with fibro that's a very individual thing. We need to stay flexible, to be open to trying new things, and to manage our routines in the ways that help us best.

Indeed, alternative therapies are very helpful for fibro. A 1992 study by Dr. Christophe Deluze and others found that acupuncture and even electo-acupuncture were the most helpful treatments available for fibromyalgia. If you are fearful of needles, though, there are many other treatments, including massage, chiropractic treatments, other body work, and supplements.

Staying "flexible" mentally may be more difficult. Fibrofog is a real thing and definitely impacts your ability to think "on your feet." However, keeping your mind sharp through various hobbies and interactions will help. Reading, crossword puzzles, Sudoku, video games, and supplements such as 120 mg a day of ginko biloba can help a great deal.

Sadly, you cannot prevent fibrofog all the time. And so, this leads to the biggest thing you must do now that you have been diagnosed with fibro: adjust your expectations.

Your life is different now. You must accept this and learn your new limitations, because you are not the person you were before you got sick. You have limitations now, and if you do not respect them you will hurt yourself. Learn your body's warning signs and pay attention to them when they crop up. Recognize that you will have days where you feel like you're underwater, where you can't do what you might have expected to be able to do before you got sick, and put off what you can. Delegation is good, too! If you have friends, family, or co-workers that can help, delegate on days you can't handle things solo, and offer help on days you're doing well.

Medications are important, too. Whether you choose to simply use Advil, Tylenol, or another over the counter medication to help your pain levels, go all-in with a prescription painkiller, or a medication like Lyrica or Savella, you will need to experiment to see what works. Medications that work are invaluable in treating fibro. If they don't work, though, all is not lost. You'll just need to develop a routine that works for you, with yoga, exercise, rest, or some other adaptation.

Living with fibromyalgia is not easy, but once you learn your personal limitations, you can work around it and maintain your quality of life.

When you resume your activities, return to work, or interact with people, you'll be asked about your illness. This is when life-with-fibro can be incredibly complicated. It isn't easy to talk about fibromyalgia in general thanks to the brain fog, but it becomes especially challenging when you're in the midst of a flare. I recommend coming up with a short, punchy description that you memorize for those tired, fogged moments when someone says "what were you diagnosed with again?"

When I am asked what's wrong with me, I generally say "I have a chronic pain condition." If they press, or say something like "what, arthritis?" then my response depends on my level of brainpower and fatigue. If I'm tired, I may simply say yes. If I'm feeling up to it, I'll say "no, it's fibromyalgia." Thanks to the commercials for Lyrica, more people are aware that fibro exists, and have a limited understanding of it.

Unfortunately, there are still myths and misinformation out there, and the commercials can't fix that. And so, when you tell someone you have fibromyalgia, you may end up having to correct their assumptions. Be prepared, just in case.

It can be worse if your family doesn't understand or accept the fibro. You may have to deal with the people you love being unwitting obstacles to your recovery. Talking to the people you love is different from talking to strangers.

You would expect them to be able to see what you're going through and thus accept it easily.

Some, however, will go into denial just as some people with fibro do. Some will accept that you are ill, but be convinced the diagnosis of fibro is wrong and thus fight with you to find another doctor, one who will diagnose you with something different. Or they'll go searching for a 'cure' and bring you all kinds of crazy things to try in order to 'fix' you. Some will accuse you of malingering, or of faking it, without realizing how cruel that is to those of us with fibro who are trying desperately to find our place in a world that has shifted beneath our feet.

Dealing with these people is draining. It is harder than dealing with strangers, because you want the people you love to support you, not inadvertently tear you apart. Most of the time, if you explain how hurtful the things they say are, they will adjust. Particularly a spouse or parent, if they love you, they don't want to hurt you. Sometimes, even just saying "I can't hear this right now, give me some time and we'll discuss it" can at least give you the time to marshal the arguments you may need to make with the loved one.

Some, however, are malicious. Whether it is because they are broken themselves, or because they are angry or hurt or feel that you've "failed" them, they will continue to badger and belittle you until you either snap (in which case they can be the hurt martyr) or cut them out of your life. I have no plan for how you deal with these people; they are a drain. I'd recommend you cut them off, but if they are your family I know sometimes you cannot. Cut back on contact with them as much as possible, particularly during times your resources are low, if you cannot cut them out of your life completely.

And seek therapy for yourself first. Add your family in if they express interest, as it can be helpful to show them constructive ways they can help you and deal with your illness. Finally, seek the company of those who are dealing with the same things you are, so that you have support from somewhere if your family proves unsupportive. You need and deserve to be uplifted while you find your new normal.

Chapter 4—Flares and how to deal with them

Fibro sufferers have to deal with the wonderful things called "flares." This is when your illness worsens, briefly, and thus you find yourself unable to cope with your day-to-day routine, sometimes completely. Flares are not fun. They are also a part of life with fibro, and so we all need to develop ways to deal with them.

There are several different ideas about how to deal with flares. Some people say to take it easy and do less. Sleep, avoid stress, and let your body do what it needs to do. Some people say to exercise gently and keep your body limber. Honestly, both of these approaches work—it depends on you, and on your flare. For severe flares, you may need to rest in the beginning and then as the flare 'dissipates,' you will be able to exercise some and help your body to shake off the rest. Medication can also help to mitigate some of the symptoms.

For other, less severe flares, you may find that stretching helps and makes you feel better from the beginning. A combination of medication and stretching can make you feel almost "normal" if your flare is particularly mild.

Some people truly cannot stand any kind of activity during a flare. For those people, resting, sleeping as long as they can, and low-key activity will be key in helping them to make their flares go away.

One of the more unusual 'treatments' that I tried was exercises involving breathing. There are various breathing exercises associated with meditation and with yoga, most notably pranayama breathing. These exercises are actually recommended to help with fibro in general, and for some people can help improve your energy levels, your pain tolerance, and your brain power as well!

My favorite breathing exercise is the "breath of life." Open your mouth, relaxing your lower jaw as you do so. Breathe in deeply through both your mouth and nose, expanding your lungs, and as you breathe out, tighten your stomach and push the breath out as you make an "aaah" sound. Do this a few times, at least three, and see if you begin to feel more alert. Another breathing exercise is to equalize the time that you breathe in and out. Breathe in, counting to yourself rhythmically as you do so, then breathe out and count. Attempt to match the in count and the out count. I use this exercise at night when I'm getting ready to fall asleep.

A final exercise is to breathe in deeply through your nose and release the breath through your mouth. This one is very good for relieving tension in the upper body.

There are other things you can do to help mitigate a flare if you have the resources. Massage and acupuncture help, though you have to be careful not to aggravate any tender points. Some people find aromatherapy to be helpful, too, though you must be careful to avoid allergens with that treatment.

Essential oils in a warm or hot bath can help a great deal. Recommended oils include basil, chamomile, lavender, sage, cypress, and neroli. Try them out individually and in combination to see what helps you the most. The thing that I find most helpful is a warm bath with salts or oils, low music, and a good book. I use various oils depending on what's bothering me, though my favorites are either mint or sage and lemongrass. Aromatherapy really does help, for me.

Also, don't discount alternative therapies like reiki and quantum touch. Sometimes the new age treatments actually work, even if the scientific community cannot tell us why.

Stress makes flares worse, so you will want to do your best to avoid stress during a flare. I know that sounds like an impossible task, but a lot of how you control stress involves your reaction to the various stressors. So, when situations make you start feeling tense, do a deep breathing exercise, or step away from and regroup. You can control your reaction to stress, and that goes a long way to helping you to deal with your flare in a constructive manner.

To "avoid" stress: eat right, sleep a reasonable amount, and avoid conflict and stressful situations. When you have to deal with stressful situations, control your reactions. Don't let yourself get angry and upset, and when you start to feel tense or frustrated, walk away. Even if the only place you have to go is the bathroom to splash water on your face, then that can help you to regain your peace of mind and control.

Another way to 'avoid' stress is to make plans. Plan for the worst case scenario, so that you are prepared if it happens. Then, don't worry about it, because you're prepared. That is easier said than done, I know, but if you can make a start, you'll reduce your own stress levels amazingly.

When you are in a flare, you may find that your mind power is not as sharp as it usually is. So, you may find yourself feeling frustrated or discouraged because of that. Try to recognize that a flare is a difficult time, and be gentle with yourself. Don't push, don't try to 'muscle' through it, and don't try to force yourself to be as sharp and as active as you are when you are not in a flare.

If you work a day job, definitely plan for the time when you are going to have a flare and still need to deal with your work. Make a list so that you can check things off as you complete them. Do 'busy work,' or paperwork that isn't detail-oriented, so that you can go line by line and see if you miss anything. Double check yourself in your usual tasks so that you don't miss anything. Also, take copious notes and check with your boss or coworkers to make sure you are clear and have got all the details right. Working with a flare isn't easy, but you can do it!

In relationships, you may need to ask your partner for greater allowances when you're in a flare. They may need to help you clean up more, or you may need to take longer doing normal chores and tasks. They may need to be more gentle with you, put off snuggling or sexual activities, or even let you sleep in a different room. It's very difficult during a flare, for the sufferer and for the partner, because your endurance changes day to day, and your tolerances are low. Some flares make people with fibro very emotional, too, and that can be hard to handle. Your partner needs to know how you're feeling so they can help. Communicate as best you can, and don't be afraid to ask for the help you need.

As mentioned earlier, during flares, you may find that your emotional resources are low. You may feel irritable, weepy, needy, or angry. You may feel that you can't deal with people, even your family. Don't push yourself. Take as much time as you can by yourself if it helps, and do what you can to make your life easier. Use freezer-dinners or ask your partner or family to make or buy dinner for everyone. If you're feeling needy, snuggle your sweetie or find a trusted friend to help you by cuddling or giving verbal reassurance. If you haven't the energy to do the cleaning or laundry or whatever, ask for help if you can't let it slide for a bit. I break tasks down when I'm in a flare. If I need to vacuum, I do one room and then rest a while, or do one room a day. I clean the kitchen while I'm heating things in the microwave, or I pull a stool in to the kitchen and sit while I do dishes. Whatever you can do to make your life easier, do it, even if it seems silly.

Use the flare as a time where you can be gentle and kind to yourself, and 'spoil' yourself a bit. Learn what works for you to help you cope. I generally need a day or so to adjust to dealing with the flare, and then after that I begin trying to mitigate it through stretching, sleep, and gentle care. Seek out the things that will help you, and use them to help make your flare shorter and more bearable.

Chapter 5—Invisible Pain

Living with fibromyalgia means walking through your days looking fine. Invisible pain is not easy to deal with because people assume you're normal when you are not. While it makes it easier for those of us with fibro and other invisible illnesses to 'pass' when we don't want to deal with being different, it also makes things more difficult, because people dismiss what they cannot see. They don't see our pain, our disability, so therefore to them it doesn't exist.

Explaining that no matter how we look, we feel horrible can be draining. It also earns us skeptical looks, and the easy dismissal of those who don't see our daily struggles. "Oh, it can't be that bad," or "well, just push through the pain," are most often heard from acquaintances, but sometimes even family or co-workers will also use these phrases to discount our problems. We can't point to a broken limb or a cut gushing blood, and we do our best to look good and act upbeat when we are out among other people, and that often makes it harder for people to see how we struggle. When we are with others, that is our time to shine, and we don't want to bring people down by being obvious about our pain, or being honest about how crappy we often feel. So, we hide the truth of our pain, and make other people even more skeptical of what we're going through.

Of course, the flipside of that is that if we are honest about how bad we feel, people don't want us around! So we are stick in a loop, a catch-22 of pain and loneliness or struggle and illusion.

It is exhausting, explaining to people without chronic pain how hard it can be for us to maintain our lives. When asked about fibro, I often give the simplest explanation possible, because I don't want to have to deal with the long, drawn-out conversation that accompanies a detailed explanation. But that can be doing a disservice to our friends and loved ones.

The people who love us do want to know what we are dealing with, and that's why I often give people who ask me about it the "Spoon Theory" written by Christine Miserandino. It is a short essay about how people with fibro have limited resources, using spoons as a metaphor for energy. (www.butyoudontlooksick.com) It illustrates very well the problems that people with fibro have in allocating their resources since even the smallest action, like showering, costs them in energy. It is much easier to hand someone a print out or send them to a website than it is to attempt a long, drawn-out explanation on your own.

If the Spoon Theory doesn't work or doesn't feel like the right thing for you, there are other ways to get across that your energy is finite despite the fact that you look fine. Explaining that for you, showering and getting dressed cost in energy can help people to see that the smallest tasks are hard for us, that they cost us more than they would a healthy person.

The biggest thing is to recruit your friends to help you, get them on your side. With good friends who understand what you're going through, you will have people to call upon when you haven't the energy to explain (again) about the fibro. Also, once good friends understand what you're going through, they will be there for you even when you're not feeling perky or upbeat. They will be better able to understand what you're going through, even if they can't always empathize.

The one thing you need to be aware of is these friends worrying about asking you to go out to various events because they know what it will cost—you will need to reinforce that you'd rather be asked and have to say no than to never know what your friends are doing, or never be invited to join them. It is hard to find a balance, sometimes, but it's worth it to maintain friendships and relationships.

Of course, you don't want to be a burden on your friends. That's never the goal, and when you're tired and your friends are helping you explain the fibro to someone who doesn't get it, it's easy to feel conflicted, happy they're supporting you and sad that they have to help. But remember that they love you and want to support you, and for some, feeling useful or needed can be a good thing. Just try to maintain a good balance, and show your appreciation as much as you can.

That is important, to show your appreciation for your friends in large and small ways. Even if it feels like you're not doing much, it can be huge to the person who receives your gift or kindness. Plus, this kind of action reinforces the friendship. It shows the person that you're aware of their support and that you value it. It doesn't have to be a monetary gift, though if you're in a good financial situation, it certainly can be. But small things matter, too. Making something for your friends is extra-special, given that you are spending precious spoons on them. Gifting them with home-made foods, hand-made goods, or even an act of kindness—helping a girlfriend dye her hair, or offering to house sit for a friend while they're out of town so they don't have to kennel their pets—any way that you can help your friends be aware of how much you value them is worthwhile. Stay alert to the ways that you can show the people you love that you appreciate them. This includes your spouse.

For many people with fibro, it's difficult to show how vulnerable they are. However, it's important that your spouse be aware of your limitations and battles while you are dealing with your illness. They can help, and if they are compassionate, they should *want* to help, so that you are not taking an undue burden upon yourself. However, this puts some of the burden upon them, and you should pay them back in the ways you can. Making a special meal, helping them organize their workspace, helping with a computer problem, dressing up for them for no reason, or serving them drinks (tea, wine, etc) in the evening can all be ways you show your mate they matter and that you appreciate them taking care of you. If you are not up to physical actions, that's ok; don't discount the importance of saying thank you. Verbal appreciation can help as well.

Of course, sometimes no matter what you do, your partner does not see it, and he or she grows apart from you. This can take many forms: resentment, anger, apathy. The end result, however, is often a parting of the ways.

It is important to examine the failure, to take what good from it you can. If it is a matter of the two of you growing apart, then it is no-fault and no-worries. If the other person grew to resent you and your limitations, you cannot change that, and need to recognize that your partner's inability to adapt is not your problem to solve. If you grew to resent the person's able-bodied ability to do what he or she wished, however, then you need to examine why. You need to recognize that unless you find a partner with fibro, you will need to deal with an able-bodied partner who can do more than you can. You need to let go of how things should be and realize that you *can* still have a happy life within your own limitations, if you are willing to adjust your expectations. Find out what you need to be happy, and make that your goal.

Finally, in the immortal words of RuPaul: "If you can't love yourself, how the hell you gonna love somebody else?"

That may sound like a cliché, but it is true. You need to love yourself despite your limitations, despite your baggage. You need to recognize that your suffering really does make you stronger, and that your uniqueness is valuable to the people who love you—fibro and all. You are in control of your own happiness. I don't mean to diminish your suffering if you have depressive disorders, but I *do* believe that you can find happiness despite it as long as you are properly medicated and you look for the positive. If you choose to look for the bad things, to dwell on the "can't" and the pain, then you will not find happiness. If you acknowledge the pain and the bad, but continue to look for the good, you'll also find it, and it will make you happier along the way.

There will always be setbacks. Continue to strive for your goals despite them, and you'll make progress. Don't let the pain keep you from your life.

Chapter 6—You and your doctor

Finding a doctor who will work with you and not simply medicate you—or worse, belittle your illness—is an important part of any fibro sufferer's life. As of this writing, there are still doctors out there who use the excuse that fibro is a "woman's disease" to dismiss it, or even believe it isn't a real illness at all. Should you run across one of these doctors in your search for your medical team, fire them! Don't let any doctor tell you that this illness is not real, or is only in your head, or that you can't possibly have fibro and it must be something else. It is real, and sufferers live with it every single day. Going through needless tests to "find the real problem" will only delay you finding the right treatments for you, and will waste precious time and energy. If your doctor wants to put you through that—especially if you've just been through it once to get this diagnosis—you probably want a different doctor. Of course, if you haven't been through all the diagnostic tests, you should allow your doctor to test you to rule out other illnesses. But don't continue to search after your diagnosis if you can help it. The tests are needless and some of them can be painful, and the stress of the pain plus the search may cause you to go into a flare.

During my search for the right medical help, I got accused of doctor shopping. I was not asking for pain medication in my interviews with doctors. I went into their offices and asked them how they'd treat fibromyalgia. I got a myriad of answers, most of which made me want to laugh or cry. I had doctors sneer at me that they didn't treat fibro, had doctors say they'd test me for other things because fibro "wasn't real," had doctors refer me to psychiatrists and rheumatologists, and had a rare few who listened and offered real help.

The ones that listen are the ones you want to keep. I know I am keeping my good doctor.

During my general practitioner search, I was fortunate in that I had an excellent mental health team. I went to a psychiatrist the first time for an unrelated issue, but he quickly became part of my "fibro team" because he listened, and when I was dealing with bad doctors, he helped me to see how their assumptions and improper behavior were wrong, and was willing to call me out if I did something that wasn't helpful in my search. My psychiatrist has helped me in myriad ways, not the least of which was reinforcing that I wanted a *good* doctor and not just any doctor. I wish that all of you could have that support. Since I know not all of you can have an awesome doctor like my psychiatrist, I am telling you what he always told me: doctors must listen to their patients or they cannot treat the actual problem. I will stress that you must find a doctor who listens.

To find said good doctor, you can do a lot of different things. I highly recommend asking around. Whether it's from friends who have fibro as well, or simply family and friends, ask about their doctors and experiences with health care. You'll likely get a lot of horror stories, but you may get some good tales, too. Pay attention. "Oh, he's an excellent doctor, but his bedside manner sucks," could mean that he'd be a great fit for you, if you have thick skin and don't need a doctor with charm or tenderness. But if you're thin-skinned and like a doctor to hold your hand, he's definitely not the one for you. On the other hand, if you hear "she's awesome, but she's always asking me if I'm ok with the treatment plan," that says perfect fit for our thin-skinned friend, but perhaps not great if you dislike fuss.

Do your homework. If you haven't found any good recommendations from friends and family, look up doctors on the internet and start calling their practices. There, you can find one of your best allies in the quest for Dr. Perfect-For-You: the office manager at the practice. The office manager will be able to answer any question you have about the doctors he or she works with, and can let you know if you fit in with the patient profile. You can ask them common sense questions that the doctor might not even know the answers to: Who handles the doctor's patients if the doctor is out sick, or would you have to reschedule your appointment? Which hospital does your doctor's practice affiliate with? The aforementioned patient profile is important, too. If the practice mainly treats seniors and you're in your 20s, this might not be the place for you. On the other hand, if the practice treats chronic pain, perhaps it's perfect for you even if the patient profile skews towards the older crowd.

Office managers are gems. If you can get on their good side, you can get their best recommendation for you—which may not be the doctor you selected! I highly recommend talking to the office manager if you can. Be polite. If they're busy, offer to leave a message for them. Be clear and concise in your message, and then be patient. Give them time to return your call; make a note that you left a message and move on to the next practice. If you find the perfect doctor, be polite and call back to let them know they can disregard your request.

Let's say you found Dr. Perfect-For-You. You've made the appointment. Now prepare yourself for it! Gather as much of your health-history as you can. This means all medications, supplements, and vitamins that you currently take, the dosages of the medications, and why you take them, all surgical procedures you've had (and dates), family medical history, current medical issues, how you're treating them, and if the treatments are still working or not. Get it into as concise a form as you can (there are great forms online that you can use for this) and be prepared to answer questions when you hand it to the doctor.

When you go in to see a doctor for the first time, it's important to arm yourself with information: both your medical history and any new information about fibromyalgia (and whatever other diseases you may need to address). New treatments are always coming out, and you want to make sure that your doctor is up to date, or is willing to do homework to help you. By bringing the information already prepared, you cut down on the time the doctor needs to spend asking questions, and you can spend that time working on answers. Also, don't discuss feelings of depression and anxiety with your primary care doctor. It's not relevant to them. You can mention that you have been depressed if you feel it's necessary, but if you can, reserve the talk of depression and anxiety for your psychiatrist. Let your doctor help you with the physical, and your psychiatrist help you with the mental.

Let's say you've been going to see Dr. Wrong for a while. He dismisses your concerns about fibro; he refuses to treat you; he insists you see a psychiatrist for fibro care (more later on why this is a bad idea).

Fire him! Respect yourself and recognize that your needs are not being met. There are a ton of doctors out there who will treat you, and who will respect you. The doctor is not god. They are human, fallible, and sometimes make mistakes. I have only fired one doctor, but his treatment of me was traumatic rather than helpful, and he broke any trust I had in him. It was not easy, and to this day I have a lot of trouble trusting doctors, but I have found another doctor that listens and cares about my health, and that's important.

We all deserve care and quality treatment. Demand that, and if you're not getting it, go elsewhere.

Previously, I mentioned that I don't think it's a good idea to get all your care from a psychiatrist. I do recommend them, because they are very helpful in helping you to know when you're being "crazy" and when you're not. If you have the depression that often accompanies fibromyalgia, having a psychiatrist who can help you to know when medication is necessary and when it's not is invaluable. If you have issues with a medical doctor, it's great to get a second opinion from an impartial medical professional, too, as I discussed earlier.

I don't think it's a good idea to get all your care from psychiatrists, though, because they rarely do hands-on physical exams, do not generally prescribe medication other than mood-modulating drugs, and they don't keep up with medical advances in an area other than their specialty. I have known a few people with fibro who tried to make do with just psychiatric care, and it doesn't work well at all for most of them. We as fibro patients need a doctor who can do more physical care than a psychiatrist generally provides.

Psychiatrists are excellent at helping you with mood issues, which we often get because of the fibro. But see your regular MD for your fibro treatment.

What about other doctors? Aside from the general practitioner and a psychiatrist, sometimes other doctors will be recommended to treat specific issues. For example, if your general practitioner isn't sure what your stomach problem is, you may be sent to a gastroenterologist for an in-depth investigation. Some doctors will refer you to a rheumatologist for fibro treatment, if they are uncertain what treatment would be best. Some doctors will refer you to a pain management specialist, particularly if you have additional pain issues aside from the fibro, like chronic back issues or arthritis.

I do not think that pain management specialists are particularly necessary, but if your general practitioner thinks they are a good idea, it is best to explore all options. And if you have an additional issue aside from the fibro, like a bulging disk, arthritis, or sciatica problems, you definitely want to explore anything that will help improve your quality of life. Plus, pain specialists tend to be more open-minded when it comes to prescribing pain medications, and meds definitely can improve our life.

However, pain medication is not the only way that we can treat our illness. Stress management is a big help, for certain, but there are also practical ways to deal with the fibro. In addition to the aforementioned pain medications like Percocet, dilaudid, and fentanyl patches, you can also look at using over the counter medications like Advil, Tylenol, and Aleve for lower pain days.

However, there's also non-medication pain relief. Dietary changes, herbs, or supplements may be very helpful for some people. Heating pads, massage therapy, acupuncture, neurostim or TENS machines, exercise, water aerobics, physical therapy, and walking are invaluable to others.

Finally, over the counter pain creams like Icy Hot or Ben-Gay can help a lot, too. Don't discount anything unless you've tried it and it doesn't work for you.

Chapter 7—You and your Family.

No one exists in a vacuum. Your illness impacts your friends and family, because they care about you, and if you're miserable, they're miserable. Whether you have a spouse or live with your parents or a roommate, they will see you at your best and worst.

If you try to hide your illness, you may succeed. But doing so will likely lead to resentment ("Why aren't they helping me?") and a feeling of isolation that will add to your depression ("I'm hurting and no one cares."). Or worse, you fall into the martyr trap, doing everything for other people and killing yourself in doing it. None of these coping methods is healthy, and if you want to better your situation, one of the first things you should do is discuss your illness and your needs with those who live with you.

This isn't an easy conversation, because you are making yourself vulnerable to them. However, if you believe that they love you, you should be willing to discuss the "hard" issues with them. Plus, there are things you can do to make the conversation easier on you all.

First, prepare yourself for it. Take some time and write down things that you need to discuss and things that you think will help. If there are things that are bothering you, add those in as well. Second, prepare your spouse/parent/significant other for the discussion. Make it clear that this is a low-key discussion, and that you aren't going to berate anyone, but you need some help with your illness, and here's how they can give you what you need, and how you want them to handle when you can't do chores or cook, when you flare, when you can't get out of bed, etc.

Try not to get upset, and if they get upset, offer a break so that you can be certain they hear and listen to you, and vice versa. Remember that you are on the same side, fighting against this illness, and everything that makes your life easier makes their life easier, too.

Fibro can be insidious and can blind us to the various ways that we're hurting the people we love. When you're depressed or hurting, it can be hard to care. But if you live with others, you are responsible to them, and to the people that care about you. In order to help them, you may need to push yourself more than you would if you lived alone. Establish routines, and use whatever way you remind yourself to make those routines stick. Whether it's a "reminder" app on your smartphone, a sticky note on your mirror, or a note on the fridge, keep track of your routines. That way it's easier to see when you're having troubles, because you and your loved ones will notice the changes. It will be especially clear if you have reminders somewhere 'public' that they can see, too.

For some, having consequences when they don't do their chores or self-care works, for others it will only irritate. Find out what works for you and implement it.

Also remember, if you have someone else helping to take care of you, that individual needs a break from time to time, too. Try to give them that when they need it. Take a vacation to visit a friend, a parent, or just to get away yourself. Even a weekend trip to visit an old friend can give your caretaker a much needed break. And travelling with fibro isn't impossible, as I'll discuss in a later chapter. Alternately, if you are not up to travel, encourage your caretaker to get away for a few days.

Also, a "break" doesn't have to mean solo travel. Sometimes, just getting out of the house can make a big difference in how you and your loved ones cope with your illness. Take a trip together, or go out to dinner, to a movie, go antiquing, something. Make sure that you don't get bogged down in the "I can'ts because of the fibro. Watch your pain levels, but don't stop living your life.

Finally, own your feelings. If you are sick, allow yourself to be sick, and take care of yourself so that you get better. When you are depressed, own it, and take steps to help yourself get out of it. Or, consult your psychiatrist or therapist if you can't break free of the depression. Even if you aren't depressed or sick, take care of yourself and do "self-checks" to see how you are emotionally and how your fibro is reacting to your routine, the weather, and all the other things that can impact fibro. Ensuring that you are aware of your body's status will keep you from overdoing it, or reacting poorly to external stimuli.

A self-check is a fairly simple process. You check to see how sore you are on any given day, check your brain to see how bad the fibrofog is, and then do a gentle stretch to see how your body feels as you move it. Once you know, you'll be able to say no if someone wants you to go on a shopping spree and you're not physically up to it. Or you will be able to say yes if you are. You will get to know how your body deals with the fibro, and you'll be able to see your good days and bad days clearly as you learn your limits and how your pain fluctuates.

Plus, your daily self-check can help you see how your exercise routine is helping. Or, if your doctor has given you a new drug, you will be able to get a good idea of whether it's improving your pain levels or not. While it is a good idea to give any new drug a month or so to work, you can usually tell within the first few weeks if it's going to work out or not. Some drugs will make an immediate difference, some will help after 10 or 14 days, some will take even longer. This depends on your chemistry and the therapeutic levels of the drug. And, of course, any side effects and how bearable they are. I've had many friends who swear that Lyrica improved their lives in immeasurable ways. For me, the side effects were horrific, and I couldn't stay on it. I found other drugs that I can use to help with the pain, and they are optional, which is something that's important to me. I like being able to take medications only when I need it, not daily.

Finding out what works for you is imperative. Keeping up with whether it's improving, maintaining, or has stopped working is also important.

Chapter 8—Living with Fibro

Living with Fibro is difficult. It requires a lot of trial and error in order to figure out what works for you, and a lot of patience while you're going through the testing process, taking various medications to see what helps, and figuring out your balance between doing too much and doing too little.

Managing fibro is a tightrope walk above a pit that can put you into bed for weeks. Fortunately, while it is a tricky walk, as you learn your limits and gain experience with it, it becomes easier. Often, one of the first things that is recommended by various well-meaning people is a change in diet.

People with fibro are often sensitive to various foods, and for those souls a diet change will make a huge difference in their pain levels. There are blood tests available for gluten intolerance, though if you are sensitive to gliadin, the test will not come up positive. The best way to see if you are aided by cutting out gluten is to cut it out. It is a huge diet change, but you will feel the changes within a few weeks if it is going to help you. There are other foods which can be triggers, most of which have similar symptoms. If you notice yourself feeling bloated, more fogged, or fatigued after a meal, it's entirely possible you have a sensitivity to one of the foods you ate. Testing for this is a long, drawn-out process, but it can be worth it in the end, because you will have more energy, less pain, and less brain fog.

Another point about diets is that for some people, eating better can help their fibro pain and energy levels. (Disclaimer: this is true for me.) For those of us with these issues, eating 'healthy' food helps boost energy and minimize pain. *It does not remove all symptoms!* But it definitely helps energy levels, which makes managing pain easier. I eat a modified diet, where I eat meat, eggs, cheese, vegetables, certain starchy foods (those without gluten), and small amounts of fruit. Most of these, I eat fresh or make myself. I don't eat processed food, flour, and I try to minimize my sugar intake (eating honey rather than sugar when I can, and trying to avoid it elsewhere). The diet has helped immensely, for me, increasing my energy and making it to where I can actually do yoga and stretching to help mitigate my pain. It is certainly worth trying, if you can afford it (which I know not everyone can). Food is fuel, and the right fuel can help. Find out what's right for you.

Speaking of food, cooking can be a pain, literally. We all need to eat, but sometimes we're so tired and sore it becomes overwhelming to think about making a meal. Which is why I will recommend, several times through this writing, that you plan meals and cook ahead of time. Freezing single portions (or larger sizes if you've a spouse or family) can be a lifesaver when you're exhausted. All you have to do is grab a meal from the freezer and reheat it.

If you've limited freezer space (like me) planning your weekly meals instead of freezing them can still make things easier. What I do is pick out several meals of varying difficulty, and then cook depending on how I'm feeling. Easy meals that I can pop into the oven get cooked on days I can't handle more, and more complicated meals get cooked on days I'm feeling good. I also use the crock pot. The crock pot is a fibro sufferer's best friend! If you don't have one, get one! They make cooking so much easier. You can gather the ingredients you need the night before, then toss them all together in the morning and forget about it until dinner time. It's a wonderful, simple way to make delicious (and healthy) dinners.

Also, do what you can to make clean up easier. I use the crock-pot liners, because that way I don't have to worry about washing the crock pot. I also use aluminum foil or parchment paper on my pans when I bake dinner or sweets. Every little thing that you can do to minimize your work will help you to hoard your precious energy.

Another huge problem for fibro sufferers is sleep. Our sleep is not restorative, due to how the disease hits us. Finding a good sleep schedule or medication that will help you sleep is crucial.

My doctors recommended that I try "sleep hygiene." I did, going to bed at the same time, starting a bedtime routine that I maintain, and doing relaxing things like reading before sleep, turning the computer off an hour before bed, etc. Unfortunately, I suffer from insomnia because of bipolar disorder, and sometimes there's nothing that will stop it. When that happens, I follow the recommendations from my doctors: get up immediately, do restful things, try to go back to bed and sleep when tired.

For most people with fibro, sleep is necessary but elusive. Sleep hygiene is helpful for some, frustrating for others. Give it a try, and if it helps, wonderful. If not, there are other options. Yoga late at night before bed can be relaxing for some. Meditation works for others. Still others require medicine. And sometimes, the only thing that works is doing something to pass the time until you're sleepy: reading, playing video games, watching TV, chatting with friends, etc. Experiment until you find your niche.

The lack of restful sleep can make pain management a difficult thing to find. Add in the fact that doctors do not generally want to prescribe pain medications for those of us with fibro, and it can be a truly headache-inducing process to try to find the right way to deal with your pain. Again, experimentation will help. This can be both experimentation with medications such as Lyrica, Tramadol, Savella, or other approved medications for fibro, and trying out exercise routines with low- or high-impact exercises. It can also include finding alternative medications or treatments that work. Acupuncture, massage, aromatherapy, and many other alternative treatments have helped people with fibro.

One often overlooked thing that can help is simply establishing a routine. Often, knowing how much energy you'll need to get through the day will help you. Waking up, you'll know if you're going to need help to get through your routine, or if you need to cut it short because you simply cannot handle it. For many fibro sufferers, this is how they get through a week working a day job: routine and a bit of planning.

The routine can also help you if you are a person who needs sleep hygiene. You'll know when you need to finish your work/chores/etc so that you can be in bed on time. And, if you have to take medications on a daily basis, having a routine can make that a very simple task, as you can work reminders into your day—take your meds every day when you do a particular task, or set a daily alarm.

Another thing that you may need if you have a day job is help with your workspace. As a person with a disability, it's important to make sure that your work area is ergonomically correct for you. And that any tasks that you physically cannot do, you have help with. If you have a desk job, request the most comfortable, adjustable chair you can find. Make sure that your keyboard is at the right height, and that you can find a comfortable level for your feet, whether that's flat on the floor or elevated. Keep a sweater around, so that you can wrap up when you need to, because many fibro people are sensitive to the cold. If you have a non-desk job, do what you can to make your work environment comfortable for yourself.

As far as home chores go, if you have a spouse, make sure they help you with things you can't do, especially if you work. Things like vacuuming can be difficult on people with fibro, because of the repetitive motion and the weight of most vacuum cleaners. (Though, admittedly, there are a lot of lighter vacuums on the market these days.) Don't be afraid to ask for help if you need it. Also, do your best to make the tasks you must do easy. If you don't have a dishwasher, doing a small amount of dishes throughout the day can be easier on you than doing one large load. I try to do the dishes for short bursts, ten minutes or less at a time. Do different tasks on different days, so you're not trying to do everything at once, especially if you have a day job. Try not to let things build up—doing a lot at once is exhausting, but small tasks throughout the week are usually manageable. (And, of course, know your limits! If you can't do something, don't.)

Finally, many people with fibro neglect self-care. Showers and baths can help with the pain, but they cost us in effort, and sometimes it's easier to skip the shower and 'save' your energy, or rush through it so that you can get on with your day. However logical this move is, I recommend that you try to take at least one day where you take extra care of yourself, even if it needs to be a weekend or day off so that you have more time and less requirements on your energy. It truly can help make you feel better. I try to take one day myself, where I take a leisurely shower, deep condition my hair, paint my nails, and whatever else I need to make myself feel good.

For fibro sufferers with children it can be completely unrealistic to take one day every week. But try to fit it in once in a while—every month or so, if you can. It will refresh you and everyone needs time for themselves! Even (perhaps especially) parents.

Taking care of housework with fibro can be a Mount Everest, especially since housework is never done. Asking for help if you have a spouse or children, trying to keep things clean rather than having to do it in one huge cleaning burst, and finding short cuts for some things can aid in keeping the energy requirement low. But sometimes you simply have to give yourself permission to let things slide. And that can be hard for many fibro sufferers, because we tend, as a whole, to be type-A perfectionists. So, do your best and give yourself permission not to be perfect.

Some things can help—as mentioned earlier, keeping your work space ergonomic can help with some pain. For housework, using a dishwasher once or twice a week rather than hand-washing dishes can help, or doing the dishes while waiting for food to cook in the microwave. Cooking a lot and freezing meals in one-serving containers, so you can microwave them also helps. Using disposable counter-wipes, vacuuming one room a day, or one level if you have a multi-story house, and other shortcuts can help to make it less the Mount Everest of housecleaning and more of a molehill.

Some days, though, particularly flare days or bad pain days, you may have to ask for help or simply rest rather than clean. I tend to schedule "days off" after dental cleanings and minor medical procedures so that I can rest without worrying about cleaning the house or work. If you have the time to do so, you may wish to do that too.

Many people with fibro are told not to do things that they love, including travel. While travel with fibro can be problematic, particularly with the new TSA rules, it is possible and entirely manageable. First of all, try to get a good night's sleep before you leave. Drink a lot of water, more than you usually would, so that you are less dehydrated by the plane. Pack lightly, or check as much as you can afford, so that you are not carting around unwieldy bags that will drag on your shoulders and back, and aggravate tender points. Pack a night or two of your medications in your carry on or purse, so that if something happens to your luggage you have some on hand. (I actually recommend packing a small carry-on with fresh underwear, a t-shirt, about three days' worth of medication, and 'essentials.' For me, essentials are my phone charger, Kindle, and occasionally my laptop or netbook, depending on why I'm traveling.)

If you are travelling alone, make sure you have arrangements to get to your hotel without delay, so that you can get settled in and relax. Generally, when travelling, it's good to give yourself the time after you arrive to rest and acclimate to your new location, without any demands from other people. If you are meeting people, let them know about the fibro, and that you will need to rest some after a full day of travel.

A note about travelling with friends: while it may seem like the "right thing" to do to put on a brave face and push yourself to be 'normal,' the only person you're hurting if you do that is you. Your friends will not know what a brave thing you did, and you will not enjoy yourself if you push too far and end up hurting. If you aren't comfortable explaining yourself in detail, simply say you can't do the things you did before ("I'm not that young anymore!"), and see what compromise you can make in the activity level they want versus what you think you can do. Sometimes, you may have to tell them to go on without you. That doesn't have to be the end of the world. Take some time for yourself while your friends go off to do whatever activity you're not up to. Enjoy the hotel tub, go swimming, read a book, wander downstairs and talk to the concierge about events or restaurants they recommend. Make sure to enjoy yourself even if you can't be with your friends all the time.

Finally, be sure if you rent a vehicle that it is a comfortable one. You may regret saving a few dollars on the economy or compact car if you end up hurting for days because it was an uncomfortable drive. Traveling with fibro is occasionally painful, but the experiences that you have with friends, family, and by yourself make it all worth it.

Exercise is another topic where people with fibro often get a lot of well-meaning, unsolicited advice. First off, do what your doctor tells you. If, for example, you are a fibro-sufferer with arthritis, they may recommend only low-key, gentle exercise such as water aerobics. This can help with both pain and flexibility, and is generally good for any fibro sufferer. It may seem silly, but it's important that your doctor knows what your level of activity is so that they can honestly help you with pain management along with any other issues that you're may be dealing with.

For some, more rigorous exercise will help keep the pain in check. Exercise can definitely help with the sleep issues, though if you have certain illnesses concurrently with the fibro, you'll need to be cautious. One thing I've noticed is that chronic fatigue syndrome makes recovering from exercise more complicated, and so it's better to plan to alternate exercise days for the most effective workout. I am sure there are other ailments that impact exercise in a similar manner, and so remain aware of your limitations as you begin your exercise program.

Talk to your doctor or health care team, and be honest. For those of us with fibro, some kind of exercise is important, but what we do varies as much as our individual body chemistry does.

Finally, something people get embarrassed discussing: Sex.

For fibro sufferers with spouses and significant others, sex can be a touchy thing. (Pun intended.) On days when the fibro sufferer is unable to handle being touched, what do you do if your partner wants sex? Well, the choices are simple: don't have sex, compromise in some way, or go full out and deal with the pain. Compromise is the name of the game when it comes to any relationship, and sex is just as important to compromise with as anything else.

The treatments given for the fibro often add to problems with sex. Antidepressants remove the sex drive, and yet not taking them can cause the pain to be worse. If you are on antidepressants and are having trouble wanting sex, try to find it in yourself to allow your partner to entice you and seduce you. For some people with fibro, adding a 'warm-up' routine including watching pornography, using different sex toys, or making foreplay longer can help. For others, you just have to schedule it and then ease into it. Try to maintain that connection, sexually. That kind of intimacy is important in relationships. If you are utterly uninterested in sex, or unable to achieve orgasm, talk to your doctor to see if an adjustment in the dosage of your medication or some other treatment might help. Finally, find your balance. You may not want sex when your partner does. If there is a compromise that you can come to, that would be best. Sex is actually good for pain; the endorphins released during sex can help lower your pain levels. Try to find the right balance for you.

One unusual suggestion that has worked for me is related to sex, in that many people like a little kink with their sex. A kinky friend of mine told me that being flogged helped her tender points, as long as it was a "thuddy" kind of flogger. That, cupping (using glass jars and fire to bring the skin up into the glass), and some other kinky activities have proven to be helpful for many fibro sufferers. Certainly the endorphins released by sex, orgasms, or kinky activities can help the pain to go away. If you're into a little spice with your sex, see if any of these activities will help you achieve arousal, lessen your pain, or even just bring some interest and intrigue back into your sex life.

Sex has a lot of baggage with it, too, and it's that baggage that can make it fraught. It's important to talk about sex, even if it is a difficult conversation. Open communication and tender compassion from the partners of fibro sufferers can make it easier and more fun for both partners. If there is something aside from the fibro preventing your intimacy: emotional baggage, worry, stress, or a past injury, talk about it. If you need help discussing it, see if you can find a therapist, a church counselor, or some other professional to help you with the 'heavy lifting' of that discussion.

Of course, there are practical considerations to be looked at, too. Pain can make sex difficult. Experiment with sexual positions, to see what works for you and what enables you to avoid tender point aggravation. For those with the available funds or space, furniture specifically designed for sex can sometimes help it to be easier, by providing a soft surface that molds to your body and helps support you without you needing to work at it. Now, granted, some sex furniture is exceedingly expensive, but if it helps, it's worth the investment.

Those with fibro often have little stamina, which makes sex difficult in both length and 'timing.' For fibro sufferers who run out of energy at the end of the day, having a spouse who works and doesn't get home until they're exhausted can mean sex becomes something relegated to the weekends, or 'special occasions' when both partners can be awake early. This kind of compromise generally works well, though it can be a little boring and predictable. Another issue that is possible is duration: if your spouse or partner lasts longer than your endurance, it can be trying to maintain enjoyment throughout. I don't recommend telling your partner this in the middle of sex! Rather, try to find a good time to discuss it outside of the bedroom. Asking your partner if you both can take a mid-sex break, offering longer foreplay so that the actual act does not last as long, or (again) experimenting with positions to find one that is comfortable for you for a longer act are all viable options if there's an incompatibility there.

Having a functional sex life is completely possible with fibro. One note I'd like to make for the partners of the sufferers: Don't assume. Never assume your spouse or partner is "not interested" simply because of the fibro, or "can't be touched" unless they specifically tell you they aren't in the mood or can't be touched right now. Ask, talk, and remember to express your love in as many ways as you can—including sex.

Chapter 9—Fibrofog

If you suffer from fibromyalgia, you are familiar with the vexing condition we call 'fibrofog.' For those who are unfamiliar with the term, it's a feeling of heaviness in your brain, of knowing a word and not being able to find it, of forgetting things, of being unable to think clearly. I have also felt like fibrofog muted my emotions and responses to things: happy things weren't as happy, sad things weren't as sad.

Many people think there is no way to combat fibrofog, but there are and the methods are remarkably simple. Staying mentally active can help. Activities such as games, crossword puzzles, reading, writing or journaling, and taking classes can help you to forge pathways in your brain that will enable you to fight the fog. Getting good sleep can help, also, since the major cause of fibrofog is lack of restful sleep. Exercise also helps by releasing endorphins and fighting the pain that accompanies fog, but it can be a double-edged sword. Too much exercise can lead to exhaustion, more pain, and more fog. Finding the right balance is tricky.

Other alternative methods that work for some sufferers include acupuncture or acupressure, meditation, and pain management. For some, the pain increases their fibrofog, and thus managing the pain can help with alleviating it.

Caffeine is something many people are told to avoid at all costs, however many fellow fibro sufferers informed me that it was invaluable to help combat fog. One person told me that one small cup of coffee could cut her fibrofog down enough for her to work, think, and generally be 'normal' despite any kind of fog-flare. Another sufferer said that the energy shots with B-vitamins and caffeine helped him get through the work day on bad brain days. So, if nothing else is working and you've cut caffeine out, perhaps give it a shot at helping you in moderation. I have used both coffee and caffeinated soda to help me with brain-fog on days when I absolutely had to be able to think clearly. I avoid it regularly, too, so smaller amounts help. One cup of coffee now helps me for nearly an entire day.

I have also been told that journaling helps, too. Something in the act of writing your thoughts out helps to clarify them and can help those connections that are firing slower to speed up. I began keeping a journal ten years ago, and I definitely think that journaling has helped me to maintain better clarity of mind.

Sometimes, of course, you'll be unable to fight the fibrofog no matter how diligent you are in your sleep habits or how much brain-work you do. I try to schedule my days so that I have time when I need it, to just be "dumb" with the fog. On those days, be gentle with yourself. Don't beat yourself up for forgetting the word for "milk," (it's happened to me!) and let your spouse or significant other know that you're doing your best, it's just a "bad fibro" day.

When you have those days at a job, it may be very difficult for you. Staying organized will help. If you have a job with a lot of fiddly details, make yourself a checklist, and keep it in a file or on your desk, so you can grab it and use it on those bad days. If your job involves a lot of contact with other people, write down the things you need to talk about with them so you don't forget. When someone comes in to ask you for something, take a second and grab a pad and pen so you can make notes. Then, go over the notes with them to make sure you have all the relevant details. These extra steps can save you trouble later. If your job is fast-paced, and your co-workers won't slow down to help you, go old-school and get a recorder so you can play conversations back and make notes later, if the job allows it. (For jobs with confidentiality issues, this may not be an option. If this is the case for you, talk to your boss to try to find another workaround, or ask human resources for assistance.) One thing that's important is that you never give up or think that it's hopeless. There are always ways around any obstacle. Talk to your human resources if you must, to get help making your job easier when you have to deal with the limitations imposed by the fibro. It is a disability, and they must help you under the Americans With Disabilities act.

Other options include keeping a notebook on your person and using it to keep notes for yourself. Many of my friends use their phone to keep notes, too, and use the calendar in their phones for tracking appointments, keeping notes, and reminders for important events.

Finally, proper nutrition can help to keep it at bay. Taking vitamins and supplements that help with 'brainpower,' and eating 'brain foods,' truly does work. (Other supplements like magnesium can help with the muscle pain, too.) Brain boosting supplements such as omega-3s, B-vitamins (especially B-12, I hear), ginko biloba, and ginseng or cat's claw can help many people as well. Experiment, and be sure to keep track of whether things help or not using self-checks and whatever tracking method works for you.

Keeping lists, staying organized, and using various tools for reminders is all well and good. But some days all you can do is keep your sense of humor and try not to beat yourself up for things that you forget. Remember, this too shall pass, and you'll have a better brain day tomorrow.

When the fibrofog is running rampant, try to stay away from things that require a lot of brainpower. Delegate, if you can, postpone if you can't. If you absolutely can't do either, break the task down into its smallest components, and double check yourself or have someone else check your work. Fibro fog is definitely a problem, but with a little planning and work, you can fight it, or even better keep it at bay with a bit of work.

Chapter 10—Fibro and ? (It's not usually an only syndrome)

Fibromyalgia doesn't usually strike in a vacuum. It seems to run with various other issues, both mental and physical. Many people with fibro have mental illnesses like depression, PTSD, bipolar, borderline personality disorder, and anxiety. To make matters worse, these ailments often have other diagnosable physical components, ranging from MS to IBS.

The most common illness that the people I spoke with had in addition to fibro was depression. A 1992 study done on people with fibro showed that 80% of the people with fibro also had depression. This seemed for many to be a reaction to the illness. Almost universally, learning that they had fibro caused people to fall into a funk as they learned to adjust to their new life. For some, their doctors medicated the depression, and they were able to struggle through their adjustments and find a happy medium. For others, their doctors did not medicate the depression, and they dealt with it in their own ways. This is not universal, but it is highly common. Learning to deal with depression is difficult—learning to deal with depression and fibro at the same time is infinitely worse.

There are, of course, people for whom depression held sway, and was the problem before they discovered they had fibro. For these people, adjusting to the fibro did not necessarily worsen their depression, it was merely concurrent. Depression is a difficult thing to deal with even for a healthy person, but those who have experience handling it seemed to deal with the fibro more adroitly than those who fell into fibro and depression at the same time.

I definitely recommend trying to find a way to deal with the depression, whether it involves therapy, medication, or a way uniquely your own. The first and most important thing is to identify your depression symptoms. For many, they don't realize how depressed they are until they begin coming out of it. A non-fibro friend who suffers from depression said she often figured out she'd been depressed only once she started enjoying things again. So, if you can identify the things that are uniform to all your depressive episodes, you can begin to treat your depression early, and perhaps head off the worst of it. If you cannot identify those things, asking for help here is definitely a good idea. Perhaps your spouse, roommate, or family can help you to see the common threads that run through your episodes. Once you have identified these, you can act quickly to treat it.

Another mental illness that seems to come along with fibro is bipolar disorder. I know because I suffer from it as well, and one of my online bipolar support groups has a relatively large subgroup that also has fibro. And sadly, some of the mood-stabilizing medications that are helpful in treating bipolar are problematic in fibro sufferers, because they cause other problems. Worse, some of the medications that treat fibro are not helpful for bipolar sufferers because of strange interactions with the brains of bipolar people. It's incredibly frustrating to try to treat one of your disorders and find that the other worsens—or vice versa. Fortunately, there are off-label medications that can help with bipolar disorder that don't seem to react too badly with the fibro. If the regular medications don't work for you, check with your doctor about the off-label treatments to see if any of those will help.

If you cannot take any medications, therapy can work to help treat bipolar disorder, in that you can learn tips and tricks for how to recognize your mood shifts. Therapy can also help you to manage your moods, and help you to retrain your brain in some ways. This is not a cure-all, nor is it as good as medication to treat the disorder, but it certainly can help some. However, the best treatment for bipolar disorder is definitely medication. Work to try to find meds that will help with the bipolar and the fibro.

PTSD, or Post-Traumatic Stress Disorder, is another illness very common among those with fibro. A psychiatrist I know speculated that fibro is likely caused by a trauma, because so many of her patients with fibro also have PTSD. PTSD is difficult to treat, and generally involves therapy, with or without medication depending on the worst symptoms that you have concurrently. Often, anxiety goes hand-in-hand with PTSD, and thus to treat it involves treating the anxiety or providing medication to aid with anxiety attacks. Definitely see a psychiatrist if you have or believe you have PTSD. They can help a great deal with this illness.

There are as many other mental issues that come with fibro as there are people with the disease. I recently had a fibro sufferer who also has Dissociative Identity Disorder tell me that everyone in her support group had fibro. I am certain that not everyone with DID has fibro, but I found that fascinating. I believe there is definitely a link between mental trauma and fibro, but I have no proof other than circumstantial evidence from speaking to fibro sufferers. I am not a scientist, but I would love to see more research on the connection there. Hopefully, someday we'll see that research. In the meantime, I can't say what everyone should do for any trauma they may have suffered. I can say if you have a mental component to your fibro, do your best to take care of it how your doctor or psychiatrist tells you. I also recommend staying on top of the latest treatments and research being done on your illness.

Another friend with fibro speculates that it is the body's reaction to long-term stresses. I have seen this speculation in a few books, and it seems to be the most logical answer to all the various symptoms and issues people with fibro suffer from. Certainly, managing stress is the most important part of many people's fibro treatments. It can help with sleep, with pain, and with fibrofog. The various ways to manage stress include meditation, yoga, therapy, adaptive therapies, breathing exercises, journaling, and aerobic exercise, among others I haven't listed.

Manage your fibro in the best way that you can. If stress seems to be a problem for you, definitely look into the aforementioned ways to reduce or manage stress. If none of those methods work, try something else! There are dozens of ways to reduce stress, and something will work for you if you keep looking. Be persistent, and find the right way for you to have a less stressful life.

Fibro sufferers can also have myriad physical illnesses concurrently with the fibro: MS, epilepsy, CFS, Lupus, TMJ, migraines, and so many others. For some of these illnesses, they will be primary and the fibro secondary. Thus, the treatment of them will be the focus of your health plan. For others, they will be secondary, and the focus of the treatment plan will be to make the fibro manageable and help you deal with it.

The most important thing for fibro sufferers with other illnesses is finding out how the fibro impacts your other ailments. Fibro can cause issues that will mask other problems— fibrofog in particular can cause issues for sufferers, because of the mental impairment. You can lose thoughts, forget things, and—worst of all—if you have an illness with a mental component (like MS or epilepsy) find yourself uncertain if a fog day is caused by fibro or by your other illness.

If the illnesses are treatable, like epilepsy or lupus, the best thing you can do for yourself is to be diligent in taking your medications and see your doctor regularly for checkups. If the illness is less treatable, then it may behoove you to try to discover which symptoms belong to which disease, and to try to treat the symptoms as you can. Pain management is important, too, and you must have a pain management plan for your illnesses, so that the fibro does not make you more miserable and unable to live life.

Fortunately, pain management plans have come a long way since I was first diagnosed. Everything from exercise to medication works to help with fibro, and once you develop a good plan and learn how these things impact your fibro, you can gain a lot of relief. It will involve a lot of trial and error, sadly, to find the right balance that works for you. But keep at it and you can have a good life despite the fibro.

No matter what illnesses bother you in addition to the fibro, you can find good treatments that will improve your quality of life.

Chapter 11—The things you can't control

Sometimes, you'll find yourself stuck in a situation that exacerbates your fibro, and you can't escape it. For those of us with fibro, it can be extremely difficult to deal with this. While occasionally, we have to "grin and bear it," other times we can find ways to mitigate the pain.

Weather is one of the most common triggers out there for fibro pain. And there's nothing we can do to stop the weather from changing. We can keep track of what types of weather bother us, and take steps to mitigate the pain when our weather triggers hit. For example, a friend of mine is super sensitive to cold snaps, so she makes sure to keep warm, turns her heat up before the cold snap hits, and if she needs it, takes a dose of her pain med. Another friend hates rain, because the barometric shifts make her joints ache. So, she keeps an eye on the weather so she knows when she may need extra time to get ready if she has errands, and keeps pain meds for those days the shifts hit extra hard. For me, the heat and barometric changes are my triggers. I do my best to stay out of super-hot weather, and when I can't avoid it, I drink water like mad. That helps a little. As to the barometric changes, I stretch more on those days, and take pain medication if needed.

Definitely keep track of the weather, learn your triggers, and then do what works for you to mitigate weather-related pain.

Other people can also be problematic in a lot of ways. The worst is well-meaning people who want what's best for you but have no idea what that is. When people tell you that you shouldn't do something that helps your fibro, like exercise, it can put you in a difficult situation. You will need to stand your ground and let them know that you are doing what is right for you. It can be exhausting. If people continue to believe they know what's best for you despite you telling them differently, you may need to adjust your interaction with them, or even cut them out of your life.

If these people are family, you may need to try other strategies to help them see that you're doing what you need to do to take care of yourself. One thing I recommend is to try to drag them with you to the doctor, so that they can hear for themselves that what you're doing is the right thing for you. Sometimes having that authority figure say it makes a difference. If you can't manage that, or if they continue to insist that you're wrong, even with the doctor's input, then the best thing you can do is to continue to do what works, and refuse to discuss it. Gently but firmly inform them that this is not open for debate, and when they try, repeat that and shut the conversation down. You and your doctor are in charge of your health, and that is the final word on your fibro.

The type of person that makes me the angriest is the well-meaning person who tries to "help" with all kinds of silly, fluffy articles on how to "deal with pain." Generally, these articles are designed for people with temporary pain issues, not someone with chronic pain. And when they are written for chronic pain sufferers, they're often so full of fluff that it's hard not to feel patronized. "Don't think about the pain" is a lovely platitude, but it's completely useless when the pain has you curled up in bed unable to move, crying because you have things you need to do but you can't get up to do them.

I haven't developed an ideal strategy for dealing with these lovely souls, because they do mean well—but often they just incite frustration, at least for me. I have tried education, gentle redirection, ignoring their messages, and—during one particularly bad flare—blowing up at them because they were a convenient target. (I *really* don't recommend that last tack. It's a waste of precious energy and you only create more problems!) For the most part, it seems that they learn over time. Most of my friends that have stuck around have gone from the aforementioned well-meaning, trying souls to people who recognize that I stay on top of my illness and try to keep up with trends and info, and that I prefer active management to passive help.

If you have well-meaning souls who are driving you insane, my recommendation is to take their help with a grain of salt, and to talk to them about how you deal with your illness. Education, here, seems to be the best route. If they persist, then you can simply ask them to stop. Hopefully, they'll listen. And if they don't listen, either ignore them or repeat to them that your health is between you and your doctor.

Other people can cause issues in so many ways. If you have food allergies, going to friend's houses can be fraught with pitfalls in the form of food that you may need to avoid. For some people, it's easy to say "I am allergic to wheat, so I can't have bread." For others, your food allergy may be unusual and so common it's nearly impossible to avoid, like corn. I have a friend with a corn allergy who, because of the severity of her allergy, simply avoids eating at other people's houses and instead holds small parties when she has the energy. For many fibro sufferers, that's not an option, but if it is, definitely put it into practice.

If your friends are understanding and willing to accommodate you, take advantage of that and enjoy their company. If they are resistant—and you'd be surprised at how many people disbelieve those of us with food allergies—then you may have to avoid their parties, or see them only in places where you can control the food you eat. It can be a mine field, but it can also be worth it. It will often show you which friends are true friends.

Relationships are often fraught with baggage, and if you're looking for a relationship and you have fibro and all the myriad issues that come with it, you may feel like you'll never find anyone. Don't let the voices in your head tell you that. There is someone out there for everyone. I recently saw a TV show about terminal illnesses, and a man spoke heartbreakingly about how he only wished he'd known his late wife before she'd gotten sick (some form of cancer, if I recall correctly). He talked about how it was an honor to help her through her illness. He met his wife when she was already sick, and loved her through the worst of it. And he is not alone, the entire show was filled with people who stood by sick spouses and significant others.

It's not easy, though, and I will freely admit that. One thing that can help is to maintain a positive outlook. I know that sounds like a platitude, but in truth, research has shown that a positive outlook helps everything—pain levels, attractiveness, etc. I'm not suggesting that you ignore or deny the pain, or pretend everything is fine if it isn't. But I am saying if you work at looking on the bright side and staying optimistic, it can make a lot of things easier and that includes finding the right person for you.

In this internet age, it's very easy to meet people online through various matchmaking sites. Indeed, after a cursory search it seems to me that there are niche sites for just about any group you might want to label yourself under, including disabled. While that won't help you go on the date, you can at least discuss your limitations with the person you're considering going out with. I do recommend being honest with any potential dates. It may feel awkward and vulnerable, but you really don't want to end up with someone who isn't willing to work with you or accommodate your limitations.

Finally, have fun! Yes, you have a chronic illness, and yes you have limitations, but that doesn't mean your life is over, or that you can't have fun. Find things that you enjoy, and that feed your spirit, and do them! I know people with fibro who horseback ride, ice skate, write, go to poetry readings, travel, and generally live their lives and are very happy despite the fibro. So don't think your life is over! It's just beginning.

There are always going to be crazy, unexpected circumstances that cause problems with your fibro. A change of job, a move, family changes via birth or death, etc. The best way to deal with these is to be gentle with yourself and give yourself the time and space to adjust. Also, keep your medications on hand, and maintain your routine as much as possible. Routines help as well, and they can also give you comfort while you adjust to all the changes.

If your change is a move, be sure to label your boxes clearly so that you can find the things you need to make the new location a comfortable home for you. Clearly labeling boxes and packing a special box with all the things you need immediately can help a great deal as you get settled in to your new home. I will discuss children and fibro in detail later, but if you are adding a new family member, be sure to give yourself time and space to adjust to the upheaval in your schedule.

Sometimes, less happy things crop up. If you have suffered a death in the family, it is important to be gentle with yourself while you grieve. Recognize that you're going to need extra time, extra comfort, and possibly medications and counseling to get through the situation. Depending on your relationship to the deceased, you're going to hurt, to grieve, to miss them and to feel keenly that absence in your life.

In the worst case scenario—losing a spouse or partner—you may have just lost your caretaker, the person who made getting through the days bearable. I spoke with a fibro sufferer who'd lost her husband, and she admitted she'd considered suicide, because between the pain and the grief, she couldn't imagine going on.

If you're at that rope's end, please, please talk to someone. If you're in the US, call 1-800-273-8255, and be honest with the person on the line. If you're outside the US, there are still resources. Find them. Don't let the grief overwhelm you. It will ease, and you will find happiness again. Give yourself the chance.

There are many changes that can be trying emotionally, but I have been told that having a child with fibro can be a very unique roller coaster. The physical changes alone are incredibly exhausting. I spoke to one mom with fibro who told me that her hips hurt so badly during her pregnancy she could barely walk, and her doctor didn't believe her because "that's natural, it's just your hips shifting into position for birth, it doesn't hurt."

Unfortunately for her, it did hurt, and the fibro support group I'm in proved to me that she is not alone. Many of the women spoke about their physical challenges: the pain of their hips, the awkwardness of their bodies, the heartburn, the inability to find a comfortable position in which to sleep, and dozens of other issues.

And all that's just during the pregnancy!

Once you have a baby, your life is forever transformed. While the baby is little, you'll have to be up every few hours to feed it, and you'll have to carry it, which can be a strain for healthy shoulders, much less people with fibro. I know healthy people with children who had trouble at first, before they got used to the demands on their bodies.

Because of this, there are people with fibro who choose to remain childless. It's a valid choice—it's one I made—but the guilt and the lack of understanding from society and family can be taxing. If this is a choice you are considering, there are resources to help. Aside from fibro support groups, where you'll find like-minded people who will support you, there are also groups called "childfree," where people both healthy and ill will talk to you about the path they are walking.

On the other hand, though, every parent I know, with fibro or without, has stated that parenting is incredibly rewarding, no matter their health issues. I know parents with fibro, with lupus, with MS, and a dozen other illnesses. They love their children, are proud of their children, and deal with the challenges of their illness with grace.

One thing that a few parents with fibro have told me is that if they knew how challenging it would be, they may have made a different choice. They stressed that this was not regret—they loved their children—but it was far harder than they'd expected, and they wished they had known how hard before they'd gotten in over their heads.

One of the fibro parents told me that her extended family—her parents and his parents—made their lives so much easier. She spoke of how her parents help by watching the child in the afternoon so she can get a nap, and how his parents take the baby one weekend a month so they can relax and sleep a bit. Her advice to people with fibro who want children was to make sure the grandparents are able to help, or to have close friends step in and help out as they can. I have to say I agree, knowing several healthy people with children whose parents help them a great deal. It is a family endeavor, and it's really helpful to have family who are willing to step in and help when you need it.

Of course, children are a lot of fun, too! Don't think it is all work and difficulty. Watching your child grow up and learn is incredibly rewarding, and being able to cut loose and play with your children is fun, too. They'll enable you to have experiences people without children will never have. So enjoy them!

Children are wonderful and rewarding, but will definitely cause some upheaval in the lives of their parents. If you have fibro, be sure you have the physical, mental, emotional, and financial resources for a baby.

Chapter 12—Disability?

Many people with fibro are happy to work. They are sick, but they'd rather stay productive. And that's wonderful. If you're one of those people, you can skip this chapter. This chapter is for the people who can't handle working anymore, who are missing too much work and are getting fired, or who have so many concurrent issues, they can't stay healthy long enough to look for a job.

For those people with fibro, work becomes impossible due to the fatigue, pain, body issues and mental problems. So, when you can't work, how do you know when to file for disability? It's not an easy question to answer, and you're likely going to need to ask yourself a few questions before you leap into that abyss of paperwork, legal jargon, and judgment.

First off, is your disability that bad? Are you able to work at all? If you can't, you're not alone, but you need to be certain in your decision, because the requirement for disability is that you are unable to work, and that you have no expectation of ever working again. Not to mention, there is a huge amount of time and effort involved in getting disability, and you have to be able to stand in front of doctors, psychiatrists, and probably a lawyer, and say "I can't work; I need this help" and have them support you in that statement in a court of law.

Second, which route are you going to take? Are you going to try to do this on your own, or will you hire a lawyer? Most Social Security Disability lawyers will work for a percentage of your judgment and only get paid when you win. Because of this, I highly recommend getting a lawyer before you start trying. Particularly if fibro is your only illness, because it can be extremely difficult to go through the court system on your own. The Disability system is designed to discourage you. You will most likely get denied at first. (The only person I ever knew who got disability on the first try was literally dying of a rare and well-documented heart disease.) Fibromyalgia is a confusing disease, and there's a lot of contradictory information out there. The Social Security system doesn't want to give disability payments to people who can't prove their illness. So, getting SSD payments for fibro is extremely difficult. However, a good lawyer can make the process much easier in many ways.

First off, lawyers will fill out the paperwork with you, and make answering some of the questions easier. They will also guide you in answering the questions so that you are not unwittingly making yourself sound healthier than you are. Secondly, when you are panicking about whether you'll ever hear from them, or get a judge to look at your case, or any of the other things that are so anxiety ridden in this process, you have someone you can call and ask "is this normal?" I only did that three times in the six year process of getting my disability settlement, but I consider my money well spent, because my lawyer was awesome and very reassuring when I needed him. Plus, the reams of paperwork that you need to fill out for disability can be exhausting. A lawyer can take at least some of that weight off your arms.

Finally, a lawyer knows the ins and outs of the judges who will be hearing your case. He will know how to approach that judge and say "this person needs the disability" so that the judge will hear him. He'll know if your judge is in a hurry because he wants to get to his golf game, or if your judge wants only the dry facts, or if your judge wants a sob story. Having a lawyer truly does grease the wheels in this kind of case.

If you're uncertain whether you want to walk down this particular path, call a lawyer and ask for a consultation. Again, this is generally free, and the lawyer can tell you your chances of getting a settlement. If you are a rare fibro-only sufferer, you may have a slim-to-none chance, and not want to get involved. If you are in need, though, there are resources out there who can help you.

If you decide you want to go through the process of getting disability, it's fairly straightforward. You apply, and fill out a mountain of paperwork detailing your experiences, what you can and can't do, and then wait. Depending on how your application is processed there may be a doctor and psychiatrist appointment through the Disability offices. Generally, your first application is denied. You then appeal, with more paperwork, more doctor appointments, and more waiting. At this point, there will definitely be a doctor appointment with a medical doctor and a psychiatrist. Then, if you are denied again, you appeal a third time. This appeal goes before a local judge, and you'll either be granted disability or denied again. I did not get denied, but from what I understand if you are denied at the judge's level, you have to reapply and begin the process anew.

I was very fortunate in that my lawyer was absolutely awesome and willing to help me help myself. My lawyer told me to write my local congressman, who was very helpful in getting me to the judge faster. (Yes, six years is fast. That's the speed of bureaucracy!) Most states have a representative in charge of their Social Security cases, and if you write your congressperson, you will likely get moved up the queue. The squeaky wheel does get the grease, in this situation.

These are all things your lawyer can help you with, and thus I highly recommend hiring a lawyer to help you.

If you file, recognize that fibro is difficult to prove and thus it is very difficult to get disability if that's your only problem. In this case, even if the fibro is the primary problem, it's good to list your litany of issues so that the judge (or the reviewers, in the preliminary application process) can see that you're sick with multiple ailments. This is the time where you want to admit and even stress how sick you are, not hide it. You also will be forced to face that you're never going to be normal and work again, if you go down this road.

For many people, admitting that they're going to be sick for the rest of their lives is traumatic all over again. You grieve as you do this, because you don't want to be sick, and you certainly don't want to be sick for the rest of your life.

So, you have to face your diagnosis all over again, and it is emotional and trying. On top of facing your limitations and the depressing reality of their permanence, you're going to have to be judged by strangers, starting with your lawyer, the faceless bureaucracy at the Social Security Disability administration, and likely your friends and family as you go through this process. And, in the end, you'll get a check that's ½, 1/3, or less what you could earn if you could work a "day job." It can be an insult to many of us because we generally had good careers before we became sick. It can also be frustrating and depressing. But, it is money and insurance, and that's important and valuable. You will need to decide if it is important and valuable enough for you to go through this particular wringer.

I am not trying to discourage you; if you need disability, you should go after it. But I am determined that you need to know what you're getting into when you begin the process. A lot of people will sugar coat it, but I have been through it. I receive a disability check every month, and I am grateful for the insurance and for the help that it provides; I am well aware, though, that I could earn more than I'm getting every month if I could work! That part is not so awesome to me, but it's the price I pay to be able to take care of myself the way that I need to in order to be the happiest and healthiest that I can be.

Was it worth it?

Yes. I would do it all over again. I don't feel as useless thanks to that check. I am able to contribute to our family's income, even if it does sometimes feel like a pittance.

Should you do it? I can't answer that. I hope I have helped you find your own answer, though.

Chapter 13—Socializing with Fibro

One of the hardest things to handle with Fibro is the fact that your energy resources are limited, and your old way of life is lost to you. We humans are social creatures (even introverts need people sometimes!) and losing the ability to wander out into the world whenever you want, enjoy the company of your friends and family, and do all the things you want to do anytime you get the urge is incredibly crushing. With the added burden of being reminded how "easy" the normal people have it when you attempt to mingle with them, it is far too easy to isolate and cut yourself off from the "real world."

We must remember that isolating ourselves can lead to a deepening or worsening of the depression that so often accompanies Fibro. So, we must cultivate people who understand, either friends with fibro or people who are willing to accept our limitations. It is important for people with fibro to get out of their houses and be reminded that they're valued, that they can have fun, and that people accept them despite their limitations.

When you socialize, be sure to give yourself extra time to get ready and to get there. If you are socializing in a low-key manner, with one or two close friends, try not to force yourself to put up a front of being fine if you aren't. Good friends will recognize that you are low on energy, and will be willing to help if you need or want it. Don't go out of your way to act upbeat and spend the extra energy that takes if you are among people who understand your limitations.

Recognize, too, if you are sick and absolutely can't go out, you don't have to and you shouldn't. Often, people with fibro are "people pleasers," and want to go no matter how poorly they feel so that they don't disappoint others. But if you are sick, you will only make yourself sicker and miserable, and you do not have the energy for that! Plus, your friends may notice and feel awkward about imposing upon you, or may be upset that you are pushing and hurting yourself for them. So, cancel if you must, and reschedule. While it's important to socialize, it's more important to maintain your health, and true friends will understand and stick around. Also, depending on what the event was, if you are worried that a friend will be upset and you can't go out, ask them to come and visit! I have several friends who make allowances for my fibro and come to see me when I'm not feeling well enough to drive to meet them, or to be seen in public. I keep a collection of good tea, and we have tea and snacks and socialize that way. I also sometimes hold parties at my house, and we play games or watch movies together. Socializing doesn't always mean going out.

While we're talking about it, the fear that if you cancel too often your friends will leave is often an insidious voice that makes us push ourselves. And, while in some cases this is true, the friends who truly value you will stick around. You must reach out to them, of course, and not simply trust to their tolerance, but you can certainly cancel when you are sick, and your true friends will recognize that you are not well and support you doing the right thing for you. Indeed, cancelling is the right thing to do for yourself, because if you go out while you are not feeling well, you risk getting sicker! There are few things worth risking that. Really, you are doing your friends a disservice if you push yourself because you're afraid they're not going to stay in your life if they know you're sick. It is not easy, but when you are feeling up to it, have a good, honest conversation with your friends about your limitations, and make sure they know that you want to go out with them, but you are not always healthy enough for it. Then, reach out to them when you're feeling good. Ask them to invite you to spur-of-the-moment events, when you can evaluate how you're feeling in that moment and then go if you're up to it. Meet them in a quite café for coffee or tea, and maintain low-key activity as often as you can.

One thing that helps me when I have no choice but to cancel is to remember that I am the only person in my friends' lives who can offer my perspective, my opinions, and my unique gift of self. They can have other friends, but there is no other 'me.' If they choose not to stick around, or drop me, or turn their backs on me, they are only denying themselves the gift of my presence. Keep that in mind, for it is true for you, too!

Naturally, when it comes to spouses and family obligations, all these rules get thrown out the window. You may have to attend a special event with your spouse, or go to a particular family member's birthday party, wedding, baptism, funeral, etc. There's no denying that sometimes these events can come at the worst possible time for us. What you can do, if you have one of these obligatory events, is to make an appearance, a token visit, and leave as early as you can politely do so. This will not save you the cost of energy expended in getting ready, but if you are sick and forcing yourself to be there and put on your 'social' face, leaving early will allow you to at least be able to reserve some energy by going home and resting.

Of course, if you are very ill, no matter how important the event is, make your excuses and stay home! No event is so imperative that you can't miss it. This may create some friction, but some tactful conversation later, and a genuine note of apology included with a gift or card can often smooth over any rough edges. Make a date to meet up somewhere, invite them over, or go to their house and get a recap of the details of the event with the friend or family member later. If there's video, ask them to bring it or offer to watch it with them. Make the effort, and you will often be rewarded.

If you are determined to be there, there are tips and tricks you can use to make certain that you spend as little energy as possible getting to your particular event. First off, buy nice clothing that is relatively uncomplicated, so that getting ready isn't difficult. If you have hand pain, avoid buttons and look for slip-on shoes, to start with. If you have skin issues, look for soft clothing that is comfortable to wear. Avoid fussy hairstyles that involve a lot of work, and for those who use it, keep your makeup simple and light. These tips can all make getting to the event less of a chore, and so you'll likely be able to socialize a bit longer. Indeed, in general these can help on the bad days—days you need to get out of your pajamas but don't have the energy to make going out an event.

If driving taxes your energy, perhaps getting a ride with another attendee, or even making a day of it and hiring a cab or driver. This can be especially important if the event is likely to be emotionally taxing, like a wedding or funeral. Also, if you get a ride with someone close to you who knows and understands the limitations the fibro places on you, they can also aid you in making sure you don't overexert yourself if they are willing. One thing that I will stress and repeat: don't shy away from asking for help! Those of us who suffer from fibro must learn to accept aid when we need it.

Other tips and tricks I've learned are more basic. Stay hydrated. Being thirsty will sap even a healthy person's energy, so it's doubly important for those of us with fibro to stay hydrated, particularly in the heat. And by 'stay hydrated,' I mean drink water. Plain water. Research has shown that other beverages don't replace the water that our cells lose. I don't mean that you have to drink only water all day—as I said earlier, you must learn what works for you and then do it—but I do recommend that you drink a glass or two of just plain water in the morning, particularly if you take vitamins, supplements, or medications, and often a glass of water before going out, especially in the summer, will help to keep you refreshed.

I also recommend that you eat before you go out, even if it's just a snack. If you find your energy levels dropping, keep high energy snacks like a baggy or pack of mixed nuts or trail mix on hand, so that you can get a quick boost by eating them.   Often, just that small bit of food will help get you through your event; or at least get you through to when you can politely leave. High energy snacks are best for this, but not necessarily high fat. Nuts, dried fruit, trail mix, beef jerky: things that pack a lot of energy into a small package are the best. These snacks will give you a powerful boost of energy and you don't have to eat a lot.

Finally, if your event happens to be a late dinner or is going to keep you up past your bedtime, take a nap. I don't recommend naps in general, as they can destroy the ability to go to sleep at bedtime. But, if naps help, then by all means take a nap. I know many people with fibro who swear by them.   For a late night, they're utterly irreplaceable. If I know I'm going to need to be out past my usual bedtime, I take a nice 30-45 minute nap, and give myself an hour or so after to wake up and be mobile again. I would generally recommend you leave yourself a bit of time to get moving and wake up fully before you have to get ready or go, but definitely don't rule napping out before any event.

One thing that is occasionally difficult to deal with is an overprotective spouse, parent, or relative. Someone who continually tells you not to do things, tries to encircle you in bubble wrap and keep you out of any situation that might be taxing. Since that can include just about any situation in the world, this can make your life shrink as your social opportunities slip away because your spouse fears you'll be overwhelmed.

You need to push back, to assure them that you are aware of your limitations and will deal with them as you need. Then you need to tell them, flat out, that they are stifling you. Even though you have a chronic condition, you still need to socialize, to enjoy your life. This is imperative, and should be non-negotiable between you and the people who are helping you. And yes, there will be times when you are overtaxing yourself, but if you are doing so as a choice, you need to let them know that you are aware you are going to pay for this, but it is worth it to you, and you are choosing to do so knowing the cost. It is your choice, don't forget that.

It can be particularly difficult to assert yourself if you are disabled (either because of the fibro or one of its accompanying illnesses), because if you cannot work, you are relying on the other person for financial security. There is a tendency among fibro sufferers to 'let' the other person take control, since they are the one providing the money. And, generally they are trying to help, but no matter how well-meaning they are, you need to set your limits for yourself. Not only because you know yourself best, but also because you need to stand on your own two feet. If something is worth your time and energy, you have the right to spend it in the ways you want.

No matter how debilitating the fibro may be, no matter how much you want to curl up, give up, ignore it, or whatever reaction you may be dealing with, you can and should take control of your life. That includes treatments, partnering with your doctor to take care of yourself, and most importantly, fun and socializing! It can be exhausting. It is definitely difficult. But it's your life, and by taking control of the fibro you'll also take control of how good that life is, and that can be both rewarding and confidence-rebuilding.

If your spouse, parent, or friend is particularly stubborn, encourage them to come with you to the doctor. Ask the doctor if it's ok for you to do whatever they're fighting you on, and then take the doctor's advice. Most doctors want people with fibro to continue to live rewarding lives, and so they encourage exercise, socializing, and even working if they believe their patient can handle it.

If, after your family member hears the doctor's advice, they continue to try to restrict your activities, there may be a different underlying problem. At that point, I'd encourage counseling, because it is a problem when one partner controls the other. If you wish to remain with this person, you need to address that problem and try to fix it together.

Another issue is the family member-in-denial. If you have spoken to your spouse or family member, informed them of your limitations, and you try to keep them in the loop, you are doing your part. If they refuse to recognize how debilitated you are, continually push you to do more than you can, or say hurtful things to you when you say you can't do something, they are an obstacle that you must deal with. For some people, this is a normal part of grief. They are upset because you are not the person you were, and they are fighting accepting these limitations which are going to make their life with you more difficult. In general, these people will eventually move forward, perhaps into the "find an answer!" part of the grief stage, or perhaps to a different stage. You cannot force them to accept you as you are until they are ready.

Unfortunately, there are some people whose denial is not part of their grief. They simply cannot accept that you are not superhuman, that you are not able to push past the pain to do whatever it is they need you to do. They are selfish, and they will not change.

If this is your spouse, you may need to leave. If you have tried to be honest with them, to show them what you need from them, to show them how badly you are hurting and that you cannot do the things you used to and they refuse to accept it and continue to refuse no matter how much you try to communicate with them, no matter what your doctor says, no matter what anyone says—you may not have a choice. For your own sanity and health, you may have to cut ties with this person.

If it is a family member, you would be wise to avoid them. If you cannot, attempt to recruit another family member to work with you to help them see the truth, or simply run interference to keep them from hurting you with their denial. Again, for some people this is only a stage, and they will come through and become an ally eventually, if you can bear to help them through their denial.

If this is not the case, if you've done everything you can to convince them of your true disability, and they simply will not accept it for whatever reason, work to disentangle yourself as much as you can. If it is, for example, a parent that you are living with, and you cannot move out because you cannot work, shift your schedule. Go to bed when they are home from work, or socialize with friends outside of the house when they are going to be home, or recruit your siblings, another parent, or friends to help you deal with them.

If it's truly unbearable, try to find a different place to live. Offer to barter housecleaning services with a friend for room and board. Or babysitting services, or whatever you think you can handle.

Alternately, if you cannot find a way out and must live with the person, seek therapy. There is often a boundary issue with people like this, where they cannot see anything but their own boundaries, and yours do not matter or exist. It is imperative to try to find a way to show them that they are not respecting you and your boundaries if you are to make a life with them in it. This generally requires outside help, in order to have someone they are not related to or in control of to show them how their behavior is impacting you and how it is not proper. Even if they refuse to go to therapy, you should, so that you can get some "self-defense" classes in the kind of verbal and emotional warfare that these people generally employ. You *can* demand that they respect your boundaries. It is not easy, but it can be done. Even if there's nothing you can do, talking to a therapist can help you maintain your sanity and your mental health.

Finally, as with all of the advice in this book, your mileage may vary. You may find you can't function after a nap or eating snacks just makes you hungrier. If you haven't tried something, give it a try, but if it doesn't work, try something else. You know your own body best.

Chapter 14—Fibro and emotions

One of the biggest issues when it comes to dealing with fibromyalgia is how interconnected people with fibro find their pain and their emotions. We all know stress makes it worse, but what I don't hear is that 'stress' includes your emotional reactions to various situations, even to some people. We all know that moving hurts, because of the physical exertion and stress to our muscles—but we don't hear about the day to day emotions and their impact on our well-being. I find that when I am dealing with PMS, the resultant hormonal emotional shifts make my fibro worse. I have bad PMS, of the sort that can have me crying at a particularly sappy commercial. So, when I'm that emotional, weepy or angry or bouncy, I find that the fibro can be worse (negative emotions) or better (positive).

I have talked to other people, who have found the same thing (though for the men I spoke to it tends to correlate more to anger). It makes sense, given that our bodies respond to our emotions—tense shoulders when we're angry, sinus pressure and swelling after crying, etc. But there isn't much research done on this particular correlation (that I could find as of this writing), and so I've been navigating these waters by feel rather than looking at other people's research.

Clearly, we can't always control our emotions. We can try. We can work on keeping our tempers, counting to ten and trying to rein in our anger, but what about happiness? Should we not allow ourselves to be ecstatic when we get good news, because it might aggravate our fibro?

In my opinion, that's no way to live.

So, what can we do? Well, as mentioned earlier, breathing exercises help. Deep breathing is proven to relax muscles, calm emotions, and has proven invaluable in helping me to maintain a zen-like calm when I needed it. But I don't always worry about it. Sometimes, I let myself feel.

There are times in life that are going to make you sad. Life is frustrating and infuriating and a great burden to carry. In those moments, we aren't going to be worrying about the fibro, we're living. And that's ok! Emotional stress is a fact of life, and what we need to do is to adjust and handle the aftermath.

And don't think that I feel the happy emotions are cake to handle. I believe happiness, too, is stressful and occasionally painful. But more to the point, I believe we can't go through life as emotionless zombies. I'm sure some people manage it, but I do not believe it's healthy. So, what you need to do is feel your emotions, but don't let them rule you.

For certain, there seem to be specific emotional triggers for some people. I have found that anger will almost always trigger pain once I'm not angry anymore. A good friend of mine invariably gets fibro-fog and headaches after crying. Another friend has found that depression will trigger horrible pain and often flares. So what do you do about that? It is impossible to avoid emotions.

One key is learning which ones impact you. If you know that anger is a trigger (like me), you can't avoid it, but you can mitigate the effects somewhat. As mentioned earlier, I use deep breathing to try to avoid getting so tense that my muscles knot up (which seems to be the primary problem). I take a muscle relaxer as early as I can, to try to mitigate some of the symptoms and loosen the tight muscles. I sometimes take a hot shower or bath, to try to calm myself and let my muscles relax.

You will need to figure out which emotions are your 'triggers' and do your best to mitigate or adjust to compensate for how they make you feel. It is not a difficult process, but it is yet another thing with which we have to deal. You may feel like it's unfair, but it is part of life with fibro.

You may also feel like there aren't any emotions that impact you. It's possible, certainly, but I would advise you to examine yourself carefully before making that determination. How do you feel after you get into an argument? Or when you are sad, do you feel the pains of fibro more acutely? How about when you're happy? How does your body feel when you're feeling joy? Is it better than your usual? Are you more likely to overextend yourself when you're happy?

These are things that it is important to consider, especially given that we are likely to pay for overexertion afterwards.

Many people will tell you, when you are emotional and hurting, that you need to go to therapy, or that you should 'talk to someone,' or that the fibro is clearly a mental or emotional disease, given how much you suffer from it, and how linked your emotions and your well-being are.

It may seem like I am being repetitive when I say "fibro is a physical illness," but it is precisely because of the aforementioned individuals that I continue to repeat myself. You will hear more than once that fibro "can't" be a physical illness for a dozen different reasons, but it is. And while there may be a mental or emotional component, the physical pain is real and must be dealt with by a medical doctor.

If you, like me, grow frustrated at people telling you it's a mental or emotional disease, do what I do: Tell them that medication helps. And not just pain medication, but medication designed to treat specific ailments, like muscle relaxers or Celebrex (which was designed to treat the inflammation of arthritis). It is sometimes enough to get people to back off. At the very least, it can make us feel better, because we know we are not crazy!

Finally, if you ever do feel overwhelmed, or like you're out of cope, do talk to someone. There are fibromyalgia support groups all across the country, and sometimes talking about the illness in a safe place with people who understand can help. We do sometimes need external validation, and to know we're not crazy. And, again, if you are beyond depressed, please talk to someone! Don't let this illness drive you to do something irrevocable.

Depression is a very real issue that we must deal with. And people will tell you that the depression isn't real, they'll tell you to "get over it," and a lot of other dismissive phrases. Be aware, it's very real. It's a part of this illness. It's one of the harder things, because often the depression will make the pain worse, which will make the depression worse.

There are things that you can and must do if you become depressed when you have fibro. First off, you must not try to 'gut it out,' or ignore it. The rates of suicide among people with chronic pain are astronomically high, and I believe that has a lot to do with the depression of it. You need to reach out to other people, to ask for help when you have this kind of pain.

Your doctor may decide you need medication, an anti-depressant, or you may simply need talk therapy, to get through a rough patch. You and your medical team can make that determination. Be sure to follow all instructions on medication if that is the route you go. And be honest with your therapist if that is the route you go.

Therapy can help. It is important to discuss what outcome you want before you start it, so that you know if you are going to simply be chatting with someone and airing out your feelings, or if you feel you need some kind of feedback or behavioral modification. Either way, don't hold back. Don't sugar coat your situation, be honest with your therapist and let them guide you to better emotional health.

Sometimes, because of the pain and the fog, it seems better to disconnect, to not feel, in order to maintain your sanity and your physical and emotional health. While this is probably effective for the short term, I don't recommend it for the long term.

Staying in touch with your emotions without letting them overwhelm you or contribute to the problem can be a tricky thing. Counseling can help, but also sometimes all you need to do is acknowledge the emotion that you're feeling, and let yourself connect with it. Too often, especially with negative emotions like sadness or anger, we refuse to admit what we're feeling, or push the emotion away, or dismiss it as juvenile. But, emotions present themselves to us for a reason, and we need to uncover that reason so that we can better manage our emotions.

For example, if you are depressed because of the pain and begin to feel angry, this can be a sign that you're moving in the right direction in your acceptance of the fibro, or that you're backsliding. You need to sit with the emotion to uncover why you're feeling the way you are feeling. By this, I mean explore the emotion, find the root of it. If you are angry, does thinking about the pain make you angrier, or is it only when you think about your caretaker or your work? If you are sad, do you grow sadder thinking about your friends, your family, or simply yourself? If it is justifiable anger because you are not being helped, that's good. That's definitely a sign that you are coming to grips with the problems you're dealing with. If it's internal anger, anger at yourself because you're depressed or because you're hurting, that's a bad sign. That's a sign that you're not dealing well, because being angry at yourself is pointless.

Staying in touch with your emotions can be powerful, too. It can enable you to get to the root of problems that you have, some that you're aware of and some that you may not consciously know. When sadness hits at the same time every year, even though you may have forgotten about the childhood trauma of losing a beloved pet, it's ingrained deeply in your subconscious. And when you sift through the pain, you may uncover that. Or, you may have body pain in a similar manner, every year, because of an injury that you suffered as a child. There are a thousand ways our bodies can hold on to memories that we thought we released. It is good to explore that, and to try to heal it as best you can.

It is not easy to live with this illness, which sometimes seems to prey on our emotions. But it is better than the alternative, to me. Remember that you are not alone in this.

Finally, one thing that people don't talk about a lot but that I think is important is that people with fibro seem to take on the emotions of those around them. We seem to feel more strongly than people without fibro, and actually feel anger or sadness or joy when people that we love are sharing their stories about these emotions with us.

As you can imagine, that empathy can cause problems for us when we're flaring, but I also believe that an "overdose" of strong emotion can cause issues. I've seen this in myself, physical reactions to other people's anger, happiness, and sadness. I feel a tightness in my chest when speaking with friends who are extremely angry or anxious, and I find myself on the verge of tears (or even actually crying) when speaking to friends who are sad. When other people's emotions wear me down, I find that helping "just one more friend" creates a feeling of heaviness in my shoulders, and I feel a physical strain in my body. I've had to cut certain friends out of my life in order to protect myself from acting as their therapist.

We must be cautious with the emotions of others, because I think that even if the emotions aren't ours, they can still create an impact in our bodies. Take care of yourself first, and then you can care for others better.

Chapter 15—Finding your way in life post-Fibro

When you live with fibro, you will find yourself making countless adjustments. Many will become second nature, to where you won't even notice them. Some, however, will require thought and planning.

When you have a job, you will need to make special allowances for the fibro. You may need to stop working and apply for disability, as I discussed earlier. You may just need to work with your Human Resources department to make adjustments in your work area or to your duties. If you're in the US, don't forget that fibromyalgia is covered under the Americans with Disabilities act. If your employer is of a certain size, they cannot refuse to make reasonable accommodations for you. There are many great resources if you need help with this process. Do not let your employer bully you into not receiving any accommodations you may need.

If you work at a desk job, answering phones or doing other clerical work, you will likely have an easier time getting the adjustments you need. Most employers are aware that an ergonomically correct workspace makes desk work more manageable for employees, and they do their best to ensure that their employees have a workspace that keeps them as pain-free as possible. Your task will be to ensure that your workspace is a comfortable, ergonomic location to enable to do your job and stay as pain-free as possible. As long as you are able to sit at your desk for your work hours, you will be able to keep working.

However, if you work retail, or outdoors, or have a more physically taxing job, you may find yourself struggling thanks to the fibro. You may need to change careers, or stop working outside, or adjust your schedule from full-time to part-time. It is possible to work with fibro, even though it can be difficult depending on your level of illness.

For example, let's say you work as a landscape designer. You're employed with a company that does actual landscaping, and before the fibro you would go out to the client's house, design a landscape for them, and then pitch in and dig holes for flowers, move rocks around, and various other physical chores associated with landscaping.

After the fibro, you continued doing these things, but you were slower. You found it harder to shovel dirt, planting flowers left you wincing in pain for days, and you began to need help up from a kneeling position. You could adjust here by not helping with some of the physical work. Switch your focus to the customers and the big picture, delegate the planting to your crew, and help only when you are needed. This may save your precious energy for other things that only you can do. If you have a physically demanding job, this is how you can adjust so that you can continue to work. Do less of the demanding physical activity, delegate some of your hard chores, or supervise rather than remaining hands on. If you cannot make these adjustments, you'll need to evaluate your health to see if you can keep up with this type of work.

Perhaps your job is primarily cerebral—a consultant who comes in to help with quality control, we'll say. And your attention to detail is suffering thanks to the fibro fog. As discussed earlier, adding a bit of caffeine in the morning can help with alertness, though if you've already got a two or three cup a day coffee habit, then more isn't likely to help.

Here, I would recommend either taking copious notes and perhaps slowing down, or doing the hard, quality-heavy work during your 'peak' brain hours, and taking the time when you are not as clear-headed to work on reports, write up notes, or talk to people. If this is an assembly-line style job, where you are having to examine physical creations for their quality, you may have to adjust the way you do your inspections, to help with the fatigue. But you can certainly keep doing this type of work with a few adjustments.

It is possible to have a career and have fibro. It's not always easy, but if you want it, you can make it happen. Look to your employer's HR department for help. If you are your own boss, make the changes you need to make in order to keep yourself in good health and working.

If you don't work, then you have it 'easier,' but it is still not easy to live with fibro. You will still need to do any mentally-intensive work during your best 'brain' hours, and do your physically exhausting tasks early, to avoid having to push yourself physically after a long day.

I highly recommend, if you don't work, that you play with your schedule, to see what works best for you. Try doing different tasks at different times and on different days to see what impacts your fibro. Experiment with shortcuts, to see what helps and what just annoys you.

If you happen to be a parent, you're aware of how hard it is to chase a child around when you are suffering with a physical disability! And you'll need to hoard your energy so that you can deal with your youngster. If the child is old enough to go to school, at least you will have the option to nap during the day. But you'll still have a lot to do, and the hours pass quickly. I definitely recommend that you develop a routine and do your best to maximize your energy, in whatever way works for you.

If you have a partner, he or she can certainly help, and you must let him or her. If you are unfortunately alone, you'll have to find a way to balance the needs of your child and your own needs. Do your best, and hopefully that will be enough.

Remember, you are disabled. This is a physical issue that you have to contend with, and you're going to need to make allowances for that. While you can push somewhat, you will eventually pay for it when you do. When you cannot do something, be honest with your child. There will be times when they don't understand, and that is hard. But they will also remember that you were always honest with them, and honor you for that. Also, if you are there for them when they need you emotionally, they will remember that, and while that is mentally taxing, it is hopefully also rewarding in its own way, too. Hoard your energy for your child, and give them your best, always.

Even if you don't have children, you may still have a spouse. How can you balance his or her needs and yours? It isn't easy, and there will be times your spouse will need to make allowances for you. But you can be there, too, in many ways. While your brainpower may be low on days you exert yourself, you can still listen. You can show you care through taking care of the house, cooking, taking care of pets if you have them, caring touches, and any other ways that your partner appreciates.

Once you help your spouse understand what it means to be a person with fibro, if he or she is a compassionate person, they will appreciate all the various things you do. If he or she doesn't understand, you need to educate them. Let them know that every little thing hurts, that every action costs you in energy, and they will understand and appreciate that your efforts are because you care.

What if your spouse is unappreciative, or is in denial? Well, as mentioned earlier, you'll need to have a talk. It will need to have an honest, bold discussion, which can be difficult. If you are one of the many people with fibro who defaults to 'people pleaser,' you may have a very hard road in standing up for yourself and telling your partner that you can't do something, or that you need more help because of your illness.

If your spouse is simply expecting too much, or if you are falling into a pattern of doing what is asked until you fall into a flare and can't get out of bed, you need to have a discussion about adjusting. You are hurting yourself, pushing until you flare, and that's neither healthy nor conducive to a happy life. Plus, unless your spouse is oblivious, he or she will eventually notice that you're constantly falling ill. Have the conversation, so that you can both agree on an equitable plan that will help you do some chores or work to show your affection for them, and yet still maintain a good balance of rest and action.

Distant family is a bit harder to deal with. They don't see you from day to day, and because fibro is so difficult to predict, you never know how you're going to feel on a given day, or what you're going to be able to do. So, it's difficult to plan things, and they may label you a flake, or a faker, or worse. (I've a friend with fibro whose aunt calls her a faker and refers to her as retarded. When I mentioned this story in one of my fibro forums, I was informed my friend's experience is not unique. Clearly, I am either very lucky in my relatives or simply oblivious to their real thoughts.) Thankfully, you hopefully don't have to deal with these people often. You can come armed with facts, or you can deflect.

I actually recommend deflecting. As I said earlier, you probably don't have to deal with these people often, and your health and well-being are more important than their education. Deflecting allows you to reserve your energy for other people and for things more worthy of spending the energy. So, when they make sarcastic remarks about your "fake" illness, replying with a smile and a "oh yes, my doctor loves it when I fake," or "oh, I know, I paid for my doctor's European vacation." Or when they make a crack about you being with your spouse just for their money, a poisonously sweet smile and an agreement, or making a joke of it ("oh yes, we're rolling in the dough!")

often disarms the disagreeable relative, or at least preserves harmony and your precious energy.

If they are the type that smiles into your face and speaks behind your back, there is even less you can do. Don't worry about it, really. Let them spew their venom and cultivate the relatives that actually care about you, who listen and are compassionate about your illness.

Often, you'll have some family drama caused by the backstabbing relative. If your family is the type to feed this drama, recognize that you'll need to separate yourself as much as you can. This type of drama is a drain, and you don't have the energy for it. If you can't separate yourself entirely, or if well-meaning and supportive relatives contact you to tell you about it, do your best to drop it when the conversations end. Thank the supporters for their help, and realize that the problem-causing relative must have a very small life to worry about yours so much.

With this type of person, living well is the best revenge.

And so, how do you live well with fibro? Cultivate good people, first off. People that you can rely on, who understand your limitations and respect your boundaries. People who are willing to help you when you're sick, who will visit you in the hospital on the rare occasion you end up there, who will be your friend and your spouse's friend. People that your spouse can talk to when they need an outlet to vent about their frustrations, but who won't try to sabotage your relationship. People, in other words, who are true friends.

You may think that I'm exaggerating the qualities of a true friend, or you may feel like I'm reaching too far in my idea of what a good friend is. I do not think I am, but if you are reading this and thinking "I don't know anyone like that," I think you have sold yourself short in your friendships. There are wonderful people out there, people who will do all of the above and then some. I am very fortunate in that I have an excellent support system, people that I have called friend for over half my life. I know how lucky I am, and I treasure every one of my friends. But I do not think I am unique. I think everyone—even people with fibro!—can and should have awesome friendships. It's not easy; friendship does take work, but it is very much worth it.

If you are currently lacking in friendships that you know you can rely on, check out local and online support groups for fibro, and see if you can meet people who share your troubles. I have found that it is very helpful to be able to contact a support group and say "I'm hurting," and not need to explain that it's a fibro thing, or justify my pain in any way. It's wonderful to have people who understand, who get it in a visceral way.

If you are not a joiner, or if you want friends who will help you get out of the house, check out groups related to your hobby. If you knit or sew, go to a local craft store and see if they have classes or meet-ups. I asked my online fibro groups about this. One lovely lady who answered is a quilter, and she attends a monthly meeting at her local Jo-Ann Fabrics, and has made several good friends. Another fibro sufferer said he took a cooking class and met a couple of people that he clicked with there. A third said that her writing group now meets at her house, because she connected so strongly with some of the members.

This kind of connection can be a godsend for you when you are feeling lonely or isolated. It is imperative for people with fibro to have hobbies and get out of the house. It's far too easy to just stay home because you're tired, hurting, or depressed. Getting out and connecting with friends or people who share your passions will cheer you up, and will remind you that there is a wide world out there that you can venture into. Plus, we are social animals. Having social time will help not only your mood, but research has shown it can also mitigate some of your pain, too.

Pets are another way to combat the depression that so often accompanies fibro. If you have something outside of yourself to take care of, often it will be enough motivation for you to get up and do things that you wouldn't do if you were alone. Plus, cats and dogs seem to know when people with fibro are hurting, and will go out of their way to offer comfort in their own (often ridiculous) ways. I have a cat that brings me glitter balls to throw for her, as though she were a retriever. And another of my cats likes to lick my feet when I'm sad.

Plus, provided you don't have allergies, dogs provide a good excuse to take walks and get out of the house, and cat-cuddles can actually help with pain. My pets are amazing, and definitely help me with all the pain and depression of fibro.

Another area that is important is spirituality. Many people find that their church and their spirituality help them a great deal. They can get socializing from the church, comfort from their pain through prayer, and support when they are ill through their fellow patrons.

Churches are definitely a good resource, and if you are a spiritual person, I highly recommend finding a good spiritual home.

If you are not a Christian, finding a spiritual home may involve some work. But there are resources, and you can find good online sites that can help you find local groups of any spiritual flavor, from Buddhist to Zoroaster.

If you are having difficulty, please investigate your local options. Particularly if you live alone and don't have pets, and your family doesn't live nearby. Look for a church, talk to your local disability office, search the internet for a group that supports your hobby. There are always options. Don't let yourself stay isolated.

Remember that no matter how bad that flare is, there are people who love you and you are valuable and important. Don't let the pain make you forget that. Branch out, find your niche, and stay as active as you can.

Living well with fibro involves managing your areas of life carefully, and putting your time and energy where you get the best reward. We've discussed job, family, friends, and social circles. I'll discuss self-worth in another chapter, because I feel that's a very important area that deserves a lot of discussion. What about time and energy? These are both finite for a person with fibro, so how do you manage them and get the most out of your day?

Well, to best manage your time, you'll need to find out when you have the most energy and brainpower. For example, for me, I don't really "wake up" until I've been out of bed for about an hour. So, I try to do mindless tasks that require energy first thing in the morning. I save my 'work' time for when I have fully awakened and am ready to get to work on mental tasks like writing, researching, reading, etc. That's generally a few hours after my alarm goes off. Then again after dinner, when food has refreshed my brain, I also reserve time for mental activity.

You may be wired differently. You may wake up feeling mentally energized, even if your body is still suffering from the fibro aches and pains, and feel groggy and exhausted after you've been awake for a few hours. You would need to schedule your day very differently from me.

There are some things that you can do to conserve energy that are universal. Schedule your day. Make a list of things you need or want to do the next day, so that you can check them off as you complete them, so you won't forget something important. You'll also know how much energy you need for each task, and thus be able to plan your day as you have the energy.

By planning your day, you can conserve your energy by 'rationing' it throughout the day. Say you have to do my typical Monday: clean litter boxes, vacuum, write a column, cook dinner and clean up after, take a walk, edit. I do the vacuuming and litter boxes (physically intensive chores) in the morning. Then I sit down for a bit and write, resting my body while I get my work out of the way. Usually by the time I'm done with my writing, it's time for my husband to come home. Depending on my energy levels, we may go for a walk together and talk about our days, or I may cook dinner and then we eat and chat. He is, fortunately, very flexible and lets me set our activity levels, since I am more likely to need to rest than he is.

Eating dinner generally refreshes me enough to clean up after I eat, and do dishes and put food away. After cleaning the kitchen, I generally settle in for more writing or editing.

Because I know my body, and I know what various tasks require in my energy, I am able to plan out my days to best allocate my time. Once you can do this as well, you'll be able to get a lot more done than you may think you can.

Chapter 16—Exercising with fibro

No matter what your pain levels are, exercise can help. From low-key yoga to high-impact weightlifting, you can find a level that will help you. Because fibro is so body-specific, you will need to test your limits and learn what works for you. No one will be able to tell you "this will help," though they can tell you what worked *for them.*

For me, walking and yoga help a great deal. I'm preparing to add circuit training and possibly weightlifting to that, but I am not going to push myself too much. I have friends who do circuit training and find it very helpful. I have friends who lift weights, too, and say that it keeps their muscles from hurting too badly. For me, right now, yoga daily and walking as often as possible (4-6 times a week) are helping me with weight loss and energy levels.

Research has shown that exercise helps with fibro. The most current research as of this writing shows improvement in mobility and pain levels when people with fibro do yoga at least 3 times a week (Fibromyalgia Network Journal). The research becomes conflicted when you add other types of exercise, and I think that's because of the individual responses to fibro. Some people will be more athletic than others, and find that more vigorous exercise helps. Others will find that it hurts, and causes them to flare.

Most people know their type. If you were athletic before you got fibro, you may want to try adding circuit training or weightlifting to your fibro routine to see if it helps you. If you were not athletic, sticking to a low-impact yoga routine with perhaps some walking or aerobics is your best bet.

The most important things are maintaining activity and improving your flexibility.

How can you do this? I recommend you start by trying a yoga routine. It is a godsend to people with fibro, in that it focuses on core strength, flexibility, and general health. It doesn't put too much stress on our joints if done properly, and it doesn't require a lot of extraneous gear. I know a lot of people who do yoga in sweat pants and t-shirts, without even a yoga mat. I use videos by Rodney Yee, because I have found his yoga routines are the perfect mix of exercise and spirituality for me. (I love his meditations; they're very helpful.) But there are online resources which are free, so you don't have to make any investment at all to start a routine. Check out YouTube for videos, or Google for instructions, and do what you feel is within your ability.

Be careful when beginning a routine, because even though yoga is low-impact, you can still hurt yourself. Don't push yourself too far in the beginning, and move slowly from stretch to stretch. Stop if you begin to feel pain, because that's a bad sign.

If 'regular' yoga is too stressful for your level of fibro, there are actually several books on yoga for the disabled. I used one when I was recovering from surgery. My book includes routines you can do while lying in bed, very gentle, almost delicate stretches, and exercises to help you recover from various injuries. It was a life-saver, and I believe it helped me recover faster.

If you feel yoga is too new age-y, you can use regular pre-exercise stretching or something like tai-chi, which focuses on breathing and slow movements. You'll need find a routine that includes stretching your whole body, and tai-chi is excellent for that. This is why I appreciate yoga, there are routines designed to hit every major muscle, and they are gentle and don't take that long. However, do what works for you.

After a time of doing exercise on a daily basis or every-other-day, you may find that you need to increase your activity levels in order to maintain or improve your fitness level. Or, you may start feeling good enough to want to increase your activity levels. Be aware of your body, and don't push too much, but certainly as you start feeling better, do what you can and what feels good.

If you fall into a flare while you are beginning your exercise program, adjust. You may want to stop exercising altogether, but I don't recommend that if you can help it. You know your body best, certainly, but if you can maintain at least your stretching routine, you may discover that you recover quicker from your flare. I definitely feel it depends on the flare, but some flares go away faster when I maintain my activity levels, and I know I sleep better when I exercise during the day.

I tend to shorten my yoga routines, doing just a basic stretch-and-breathing routine, but I have found that the more I work through the flares, the better I feel.

There can definitely be a 'backlash' to exercise. Your body may hurt more as you begin your routine. You may fall into a flare. Gently pushing through the fibro pain can be difficult. Also, it can sometimes be hard to know the difference between the pain of fibro muscles reacting to a new routine or the pain of a muscle strain.

Always stop if you feel a sharp pain during exercise. You'll usually know if you hurt yourself; there's nothing like the shock of actual injury. Fibro pain tends to be a more all-over ache, whereas injury pain is sudden, sharp, and usually brings with it heat and swelling.

Push through the sore, all-over body pain, but stop if you feel an injury.

One thing that I have not seen discussed as much when it comes to exercise and fibro is how much it can lift your mood. The endorphins can help to make you happier, plus reconnecting with your body through movement can help to mitigate some of the anger and resentment that we sometimes feel about our body's "betrayal."

Being diagnosed with fibro led to me feeling a lot of anger at my body, and feeling like it 'failed' me. Yoga, walking, and the deep breathing exercises that I began to do helped me to reconnect with my body in a positive way. Listening to it when I did the stretching, feeling the difference between the burn of fibro pain and the burn of post-exercise fatigue, and feeling it become stronger over the months truly helped me to appreciate it again. My moods improved, I stopped feeling betrayed, and I began to find joy in physical activity in a way I didn't think I ever would again. I thought I was alone in this, but another person posted in the fibro forum, asking how she could get over her anger at her body, and multiple people chimed in, stating their anger and frustration. I wrote about my experience with exercise, and people have responded positively to that suggestion. It helps to connect with our bodies, to have the positive feedback.

Give yourself a chance to find joy in exercise, too. It may seem like a silly idea, but between the improvements in your health it can give you, and the alleviation of some of your pain, exercise really can help you to be happier.

That said, exercise isn't going to fix the fibro. And it's not going to be the perfect solution for everyone. If you are able, though, give it a try and hopefully it will help.

One thing that I find is nearly universal when it comes to exercise is the fear of pushing too much. As I mentioned earlier, there's a huge difference between the normal 'burn' of fatigue and the pain of injury. If you are fearful of hurting yourself, you can often find an intro yoga class that is free, or perhaps sign up for a month-to-month gym, and see if they offer a free trainer session. Or even get a trainer to come to your house for a free consultation. And if you are worried about hurting yourself, that's what I recommend: find a way to try exercising in a supervised environment.

Some gyms offer free classes with membership, and you can sign up to try them out to see if they work for you. If you're worried about a long-term contract, see if they have a program where you can cancel within a certain time frame without incurring a penalty. Most gyms do, and it's usually between 30 and 90 days. If your local gym doesn't offer classes, check and see if there's a yoga studio or instructor in your area, and ask if they have a "trial" class, where you can go and try it out once or twice to see if it works for you. Some places will let you pay for one class, too, just to try it out.

Check around! You might be surprised at what resources you have.

Chapter 17—Self-Worth and Fibro

One of the hardest things about having fibro is internal. Many people with fibro feel that they are 'ruined' or somehow less of a person because they are sick. Add in that many people with fibro have to stop working, and the self-esteem issues become all the greater. Our society tends to value people based on what they can do or what income they make, and people with fibro often can't do what they chose as their careers, and thus have less income.

While I am more focused on the improvements we can make to our health, I'd be remiss if I didn't address this. It's a fallacy, but it's pervasive, and I believe we can combat it if we try.

First off, if you are one of the many people with fibro who had to give up their chosen career, realize that you are more than what you do. Your value is not only in your job. Realize, too, that while you may not be able to continue your career, you can earn money in other ways. I have friends with fibro who have opened stores on Etsy and Ebay to bring in income, and while they may not be making the thousands per month that they used to, they all seem happier doing what they love and making a bit of money in a creative manner.

If you have a hobby that you enjoyed before, see if you can turn it into an income. Pottery, knitting, and writing are all ways to bring in an income without working a 9-5 job, and because they are creative they can bring joy while they bring money! Even gardening can bring in income if you sell your plants or veggies at a local farmer's market. Don't discount any options; be creative.

Still, this is not going to bring a huge income, and if you were making thousands a week at a high-powered career, you may feel the sting of how far you've fallen. Realize that money is not everything, and it is certainly a poor way to value people. While you can mourn your previous income, and the job (if you loved it), don't consider yourself devalued or broken.

We have a disability. It is not the total of our lives. We are still able to be good parents, good friends, good children, and good people. While we may have new limitations that we did not have before, we are still valuable and worthy.

Many people with fibro attempt to adjust by super-normalizing, trying to prove that they can do everything they did before the fibro, and sometimes adding more. Super-normalizing is a psychological phrase, usually used for type-A personalities who continue to be determined to live a normal life after a trauma or injury. Many people with fibro fall into this trap. It generally leads to a vicious cycle of doing all that they used to do, either at work or at home, and eventually crashing into a flare that puts them into bed for days and sometimes weeks at a time. I am very familiar with this particular coping mechanism because I still fall into it from time to time. I work very hard at trying to manage my illness the "right" way, but sometimes it's easier to just try to be normal. This tends to happen at the worst times, too. And forget it if there's a vacation or special event I want to go to! I can't help but try to be 'normal' so that I can enjoy my time at a convention or on vacation.

We pay for the super-normalizing, though, because we are not normal. We need to manage our illness, and that can be a huge self-esteem killer.

One way to combat this is to remember that despite the illness you may suffer with, you are still valuable for your perspective, for your outlook, for your opinion, and the other things that only you can provide. If you are a parent, you are valuable to your child, because you are the only parent they are going to get! If you are a spouse, you are valuable for the time and effort that you put into your relationship, and for the comfort and solace that you provide your partner. If you are a friend, you can be the best friend that another person has just by saying the right thing at the right time, or being there when no one else is.

Often, we overlook the fact that we are very good at listening and being there for our friends, because we so often can't do active things with other people. If you put effort into it, you can be an irreplaceable confidant for people who need an ear. By developing other skills, things you may have overlooked when you were healthy, you can improve your self-esteem and provide comfort for other people.

Of course, this doesn't fix the fact that many people feel 'ruined' when they are diagnosed with a chronic illness like fibro. The road to combat those feelings is long, difficult, and full of switchbacks and backtracking and moments where you're convinced you're never going to get off it.

I've been there, myself. I get so angry at my body sometimes, when it fails me because of the fibro, that I end up sabotaging my progress in ways that I know aren't helpful. Still, we are *not* ruined. We really aren't. We have to adapt and learn to be flexible and explore our new limitations, but we can still live fulfilling, rich, rewarding lives. They may not be the lives we envisioned, but they can be better than we imagined if we let ourselves try.

If you are feeling ruined, angry, sad, or frustrated, allow yourself to feel that way! Don't beat yourself up for having negative emotions, because they are valid. Too often, we want everything to be happy and nice, and sometimes you just have to allow the bad emotions to come in, and work to get away from them later. So, if you're having a day where you're just angry at everything, let yourself feel that, be mad, and wait to see if tomorrow will be a better day. Most of the time it will be.

If it's a flare that's frustrating you, and you remain angry, frustrated, or sad during the flare, again, don't try to squelch your emotions. Just work to not take them out on other people, and wait for the storm to pass.

As to feeling ruined, those feelings will happen. Continue to tell yourself you're not ruined, and focus on getting through the bad moments. Let your friends help pull you out of the funk if they offer or attempt to, and work through it how you can.

Another thing that many people deal with is guilt over the disability, or over having to take social security disability income instead of a job. First off, feeling guilty over something where you have no control is silly. You are disabled. You didn't ask for the disability; it simply happened. When you feel guilty over that you're wasting your time and energy, which are precious and limited. Feeling guilty over having to take SSI payments is also silly; they are there to help you provide for yourself when you can't work. Don't waste your energy on pointless emotions like guilt.

I know this is generally easier said than done, but if you can find ways to avert the negative thoughts, I recommend that. Remind yourself that you wouldn't do this if you didn't need it, that it's there to help, and, even if you need to lie to yourself, you can always say that it's only temporary! It may be, too, if you're able to find a job that you can do despite your fibro.

Indeed, if you are determined that you must work, social security can help you with adaptive training and job placement, too. So if you are on disability, look into those programs to see if you can find a good job that will help you to earn a living wage. Or, you can look into jobs you think you could do even with the disability, and then see what kind of training is available to help you acquire one of those jobs through Social Security. Currently, there are a lot of job training programs available to help people displaced through the economic downturn, so there may be help out there for you if you ask about it.

If you cannot find the help you need from social security, there are also job training and job placement fairs, which you could look into to see what fits your needs. Colleges are great places to investigate a new career, too. Finally, ask around. There are people who work from home that can give you leads to see if these jobs are right for you. Don't discount any source if you are looking for a "real" job. They are out there, but they're sometimes hard to find.

Speaking of colleges, if you're disabled but wanting to work at a real job and not go on disability, you can go to school. Particularly if can't bring yourself to try to find a job while you're coping with your illness, school may be just the thing for you. It can be a good way to find out if you'll be able to manage a regular schedule for a short amount of time, too. You can take a few classes, even experiment to see what really piques your interest. If you can't handle a light class schedule, then you know for sure you need to apply for disability. And if you can handle the schedule, then you can get a degree and go back to work!

It is an option to explore, certainly. That's something that many people with fibro feel they have lost—their options. But there *are* options, you just have to be flexible in order to find them.

Speaking of losses, this is something that is often difficult to deal with for anyone, and it is something that we have to deal with over and over again as we discover things we can no longer do. As we go through our lives, we will learn our limitations and have to give up hobbies, jobs, and many other things that we valued. Each of these is a separate loss, and may cause the feelings of grief and anger that are part and parcel of dealing with loss.

These smaller losses sometimes add up, but they should be honored no matter how big or small they are. We need to respect the losses, and allow ourselves to sit with these feelings. Don't turn away from feelings of anger, sadness, or grief. These are difficult to deal with, but as a person with fibro you will need to learn how best to deal with them, and hone your coping skills.

Coping skills are valuable, especially for us. And while most of the books and literature on coping with loss are about losing people to death, there are still valuable things to be learned from them. Read books, talk to people, implement the things that work for you, and adapt to the new life you're leading.

Finally, another issue that people with fibro end up battling is their own tendency to want to please other people. Now, not all fibro people have this, so if you are one who doesn't mind saying no, and doesn't have an issue when people are upset or disappointed in you, skip this. But, if you're one of the many people with fibro who has this issue, listen up!

We must drill into our heads that we cannot please everyone. Write it down, repeat it to yourself, whatever you need to do in order get through to yourself. Trying to please everyone will only hurt us, because we'll go and go and go until we crash. We must set boundaries, and we must firmly stand behind them. We must learn to say 'no' when people ask us to events or to do activities that are going to exhaust us or push us into flares.

It is not easy, I admit that. You may have to repeat yourself. You may have to deal with a lot of guilt and worry that people will leave you if you don't push yourself for them. But remember, you must live in your body. Ask yourself if the person that is pushing you to do something that is going to hurt you is aware of how much you'll be sacrificing if you do what they're asking you to do. If they aren't, discuss it with them. Let them know that what they're asking you is a huge deal for you, and while you'd love to, you need to hoard your energy. If they continue pressing, remember that you can and should say no. Tell them "no, I'm sorry, I can't." Then, repeat that. If they still persist, end the conversation. If they insist that you're the only person that can do it, reject that notion, and (if you can) suggest someone else. Even if you can't suggest someone else, firmly tell them "I cannot, you will have to find someone else."

I've a dear friend whose mother has fibro, and she's the ultimate people pleaser. She was recently roped into helping decorate for an event at her church. She ended up doing 90% of the work, and was bedridden the next day. This is not the first time I've seen something like this happen to her, and it never fails to make me so angry on her behalf, because she's an awesome person. But she needs the same lessons that I needed when I was first diagnosed: assertiveness training!

I, too, used to do everything for everyone, and pay for it for days, sometimes weeks after. I have gotten better, but I had to have my therapist help me with role playing and other things that sound silly, but really do help.

If you're a person who has these problems, I highly recommend therapy or asking a good friend to role play with you, and try to bully you into something. Practicing saying no really does make the actual moment easier. And you don't have to be rude (though, you can be if it comes to that). Saying "no, I'm sorry," or "thank you for thinking of me, but no," is often more effective than being rude, though that does depend on the person and the situation.

The biggest thing you must do is set boundaries for yourself, and then respect them. It's very easy to say "just this once," and then find yourself roped into something for the fourteenth time. It is much easier if you say "I am not going to volunteer ever again," and then when an opportunity comes up, don't! When someone tries to recruit you, say no.

No is a powerful word, and you must remember that you have the right to say no at any time. Learning to say no might be hard, but it's one of the tools you need to use to manage your fibromyalgia. Part of managing this illness is using your energy for the things you want and need to do, and not letting yourself be roped into things that will tax you unnecessarily. Remember to say no when you need to rest. And say yes when you have the energy and are going to enjoy the task that you're being asked to do.

Setting boundaries, respecting yourself, and honoring your own needs will improve your self-worth as you struggle against this disease.

Chapter 18—The Caretaker's Point of View

I am not a caretaker, so for this chapter I did a lot of talking with my husband and other people who live with fibro sufferers. But one of the most common things that came up was caretakers wanting to know what they can do to help the person they love who has fibro. So, we'll begin there.

First off, communication is imperative. Caretakers need to be willing to ask their loved ones how they're feeling, and sometimes draw out their feelings. Too often, we don't like to dwell on our feelings, on how badly we are doing, or look too closely at it if we're doing well. Asking "how are you doing?" may not be specific enough, too. Rather, ask "what are your pain levels like today?" because that forces us to actually think about it. It also shows that you want specifics, rather than a platitude.

Plus, when you, the caretakers, are looking at the to-do list, ask your loved one "do you have the energy for this?" Making sure that your loved one with fibro has the energy for their list of tasks is going above and beyond in a good way. Be understanding and gentle, and don't be afraid to talk to your loved one about the things that they want to accomplish. Also, be sure to prioritize the list, so they can postpone things if they need.

In general, we like to do for ourselves despite the pain, and sometimes *to* spite it. We may push a bit in order to be able to do everything, but it's worth it in the feeling of accomplishment and normalcy. But if we're sick, you may find yourself needing to help us a lot. We may be angry or embarrassed at the level of help we need, and thus not be as outwardly grateful as you might wish. Trust me, we appreciate it.

When I had surgery, I had to ask my husband for help to the bathroom the first few days. That was horribly embarrassing to me, but his compassion showed me how much he cares about me. I felt loved, and I still think of that moment with fondness. I was a cranky, unappreciative patient—until later, when I was feeling better and could see more clearly how he'd sweetly helped me. And I was certain to thank him for it!

Sometimes, asking us what help we need is overwhelming, though. Other times, we don't want to think about it. So, what can you do that is helpful without needing to ask?

Fibro sufferers tend to be cold, so making sure we have blankets available is a good thing. Warm, comfortable, soft clothing is also important. Too often, our skin is sensitive, and so harsh clothing is almost painful to wear. T-shirts and pajama pants that are made of ultra-soft cotton or an exceptionally soft blend can be worn to rags by fibro sufferers. Something often overlooked is socks. A lot of sock materials are harsh and uncomfortable. Finding soft and comfy socks can be difficult for fibro sufferers with sensitive feet. A gift of fluffy, extra soft socks is one that many fibro sufferers will treasure.

Gentle encouragement for the fibro sufferer to move, to go for a slow, short walk or to do a yoga routine can be helpful. In some cases, staying in bed can actually hurt, and asking him or her to come with you on a walk at their pace can be a good pick-me-up. It gets them out of the house, and can refresh them if the pain isn't too taxing.

Some days just quiet company is amazing to those of us with fibro. Just sitting in the same room while we read or watch TV like 'normal' people can be a wonderful change of pace. And along those lines, making sure we have books, music, TV shows, or movies we like in the house, so that we don't have to go far for entertainment shows that you care and that you want us to be happy.

For me, it's important that I take my meds without reminders, but everyone is different. If your fibro sufferer feels loved and reassured having you remind him or her to take medications, then by all means give a gentle reminder. And even I have to be reminded from time to time to take the pain-relieving medications I use, so keep an eye out for good times to ask your loved one if they've taken their pain medication, or if they need to use it for this particular pain.

Finding a good balance between concern and smothering can be difficult, but with a little practice and some good communication between you and your partner, you can do it. If they ask you to back off, do so. Always respect their boundaries, and listen to them.

Many fibro sufferers are emotional about their illness. Their caretaker will have to deal with the fibro sufferer's depression, anger, and grief while also having to handle their own emotions about their loved one's illness. This can be difficult, and the difficulty can be exacerbated if the caretaker is prone to pushing their emotions aside or being overly emotional. Either reaction is likely to create a problem for the fibro sufferer, in that he or she will suddenly be having to help the caretaker with their emotions, or worrying that the caretaker isn't able to handle this because of their cold attitude.

The best way to handle any emotional difficulty is to discuss it in a calm, open manner. Airing out the worst of the emotions can prevent a storm later, and can bring caretaker and fibro sufferer closer together. The shared experience of having to deal with this intrusive and painful illness can be a bonding experience if both people are willing to open up about their feelings and have these vulnerable discussions. Plus, if you remember that you both are in it together, and the fibro is "the enemy," this will go a long way towards helping your relationship be stronger.

Of course, some people don't like to have that kind of discussion, or don't feel good opening up that much. And it can be a burden at points, which is why therapy is always a good, viable option. Having an outside perspective, and having someone outside of the caretaker dynamic to talk to can be powerful and helpful. If you cannot afford therapy, talk to a trusted clergy member, or seek help from the many free clinics throughout the country.

For the caretakers, it's important to remember that the emotions associated with fibro can be difficult to handle. For some of the storms, you just will need to ride it out, to allow your partner or family to be angry or sad or grieving, and be there for them if they need you. For other emotions, or for dangerous depressions, you'll need to comfort them, and sometimes to bully them into taking care of themselves or getting help. For some depressions, the best way to get through them is to get up and get moving, for others, you will need actual medical intervention and a doctor's help.

It is not always easy to know the difference. Too often, the pain of fibro leads to those suffering from it needing to stay in bed. Talking can help. If your fibro sufferer is unwilling or unable to even talk to you, it's likely that a bad depression has them in its grip, and they need comfort and possibly help to get back on their feet. If they're willing to talk, but unwilling or unable to do well-loved activities, it's more likely pain keeping them in bed, and you will need to help them with pain management before you can assess their mental or emotional state.

A common thread among fibro sufferers is anger at their illness and the perception of weakness that comes with it. Sometimes, that anger gets taken out on other people, and if you're a caretaker, you may end up being the recipient of some of that anger. It will be difficult, but the best thing you can do is recognize that it's not really about you, and let it roll off your back. Engaging will only lead to a blow-up that could be bad for everyone involved. Let them blow up, and speak to them about it later, after everyone has calmed down. Most likely, they'll be embarrassed and apologetic. And if they aren't, they should be, and you can have a discussion with them about it. Remind them that you are on their side, and that their anger is misplaced when directed at you—but not in the moment. Let them have their angry moment. Sometimes it's necessary.

Another issue that you will have to deal with as a caretaker is setbacks. Flares, injuries, illnesses, all of these things can cause a fibro sufferer to go from being able to get up and do all the things they want to do to being bedridden or worse.

For some caretakers, the initial desire when a fibro sufferer hits a setback is to try to fix it. Clearly, they won't be able to magically wave a wand and make their loved one well. But there are some things they can do to make it easier on their loved one. First off, provide the comforts I listed earlier. Make sure that their loved one has distractions—books, TV, video games, internet, whatever flavor of distraction they find most engaging—and every day comforts like food, drink, blankets, and medications.

If it's a finite setback, like a broken bone, where they will be back to 'normal' in a particular time frame, it can be helpful to remind them that it will be over on whatever date they're getting their cast off. Even if it doesn't have a particular end date, reminding them "this, too, shall pass" can be comforting. If it's an emotional setback, like the previously touched-upon anger or frustration or depression, comfort is key. Being there, listening when they need to vent, and reassuring them that you're there for the long haul will help them to feel better. Sometimes they will just need to be left alone, and that's ok too.

Establishing intimacy can also help. Doing things for your partner like massage, or getting into the shower or tub with them and washing their hair, gentle and restorative things. And yes, sex falls into this category! If your partner is up for it, the gentle massage can lead to other intimate activities and that can help lift their emotions by re-affirming the connection, and boosting their mood through endorphins.

Finally, if the setback is related to emotional issues, it can be surprising how physically impactful this can be. You'd expect that emotional issues would be less physically taxing, but with fibro the emotions and the body are so tied together, it can often be one and the same. Don't belittle their emotions and the physical reactions they are experiencing. Again, offer comfort, validate them when they need validation, and support them getting the help they need if they need outside aid.

Mental issues, particularly fibrofog, can make this illness more difficult for the caretakers because the fibro sufferer sometimes cannot put into words what they need. They simply don't have the brainpower for it. This is especially true in a fibro flare, because the fibro fog will claim all mental power. Try not to express the frustration that you may feel at their inability to speak about what they need. This will only make things worse; they feel horrible about their lack of communication right now, too. What you need to do is to be gentle, supportive, and don't pressure them.

Pressuring them or putting them on the spot while they are engulfed in fog can lead to snappish responses, tears, or frustration and depression. It's difficult enough for those of us with fibro to live inside our own heads, but when demands from the outside become difficult, we tend to react badly. Again, asking specific questions ("do you need something to drink?" versus "can I get you anything?"), offering what you are having ("I was going to make some dinner, are you hungry?" "I was thinking of going for a walk, are you up to joining me?" "I was heading to the store, would you like some more of your favorite drink?" etc), and ensuring they have comforts nearby is extremely helpful and comforting.

For some people with fibro, too much information costs them in energy. They may seem short or frustrated when they ask you to get to the point, but in truth they just want to know what the important bits are. Letting them know they don't need to do anything with the information can lead to a greater willingness to listen, but if they're tired enough or fogged enough, they may simply not be able to handle too much conversation. Try to keep your conversations short unless they express an interest in talking, and be understanding if they simply don't have the energy to converse at that moment.

For the caretaker, the biggest issue can be handling their own stress at having a loved one with a chronic painful disease. They know that putting that responsibility on the disabled person isn't helpful for either of them, and yet if they don't have a good support system, finding a way to handle their stress can be frustrating and stressful in and of itself! Good suggestions courtesy of caretakers I know include exercise, getting out of the house, hobbies, and social visits.

Exercise is a good idea, anyway. The fibro sufferer may not be able to exercise as much as you can, though. So, if you need to burn off some steam, heading out to the gym, going for a run or bike ride, or even taking an aerobics class can be good ways for you to manage your stress without putting a burden on the fibro sufferer. Certainly, if you are stressed, getting out of the house for a walk and sweating a bit can help with that, and it's a good idea to get away from the fibro sufferer, particularly if they're the source of some of your stress. Going out, exercising, and coming back home with a clear head can also help you to learn the true issue you have, when you have a problem, and then you can speak to the fibro sufferer about it in a clearer manner. Sweat can lead to good insights, and that is helpful for you both.

You don't always have to sweat when you get out of the house, though! While it may seem rude, if your fibro sufferer is hurting and you want to go to a movie, you can and should. If they aren't up to going with you, pick a movie you want to see that they aren't interested in and go to it. Go grocery shopping, and pick up a few things for your loved one while you're out. Or go shopping for other things, taking a day at the mall. Sometimes getting out and doing things for yourself can really help your mood.

While it may seem silly, something like a spa day can be good for a caretaker of either gender. A massage, a manicure, a pedicure, or even just a nice haircut and a bit of pampering can give a caretaker the energy they need to return to their duties with a light heart. Be open-minded, and explore your options for pampering and enjoyment.

Hobbies are really important. My husband is a woodworker. He builds everything: from an incredibly awesome cat tree for our kitties to a sturdy and useful end-table and countless things in between! If you are taking care of a fibro sufferer, it's very important that you have your time, too. My husband escapes to the garage, and because it's a hobby he enjoys, I don't have the hyper-awareness about why he's out there. We fibro sufferers do worry that you wander off because you're upset or frustrated or angry at us. So knowing that this is something he does for fun helps put my mind at ease, because he's enjoying his time and I'm not 'at fault.' For caretakers, a hobby that's just yours is important for your peace of mind and ours.

Computers are a common hobby, but because that may not take you away from your fibro sufferer, you may want to find one that will take you out of the house as well. Working on cars, woodworking like my husband, beekeeping, pen-and-paper gaming, and sports are all good ways to get out of the house and enjoy yourself.

Social time is important. Plus, if you have friends who aren't connected with the fibro sufferer in your life, they can offer a different perspective, one unclouded by worry over the fibro sufferer's feelings. It's important that they respect your relationship with the disabled person— sometimes people being protective can be destructive to relationships. But if they respect that, for you to be able to get out and get away from your responsibilities can be very relaxing and helpful. And being around 'normal' people can be refreshing.

Plus, it's good to have a place that can be a refuge for you. Good friends are important, and a guy's or girl's day out with friends, where you can just be yourself, can refresh you and let you return to your 'duties' as caretaker with a much happier and lighter spirit.

An important thing for caretakers is *how* to take a break. It's not easy to break away when you are the main support for a person with a disability. For short breaks, clearly it's not as much of a problem, but if you want to take a longer break, your loved one with fibro might be scared by you leaving, or feel abandoned, or left out.

It is important that you take a break when you need it, even if your loved one is upset by this. They may be unhappy, but they will appreciate you returning refreshed and happier yourself. Don't neglect your own self-care for your loved one. That helps no one.

I don't have universal advice, because every fibro sufferer is different. If someone with fibro is exceedingly dependent upon you, it may be difficult to tear yourself way without tears and anger. (For the record, this is not healthy, and you should seek therapy to ensure that you are not enmeshed in an unhealthy way.) However, in general, the best way is to give them as much of a head's up as you can. For many fibro sufferers, upheaval in the schedule is stressful and worrisome. The longer they have to prepare, the better able they are to handle the disruption.

For some fibro sufferers, they'll want to know what you're planning, especially if you're going away for a few days or longer. For others, they won't want to hear about the trip because they fear being jealous or sad that they can't join you. Talk with your loved one and respect their wishes. Naturally, once you're home, the worry about envy won't be as prevalent, and hopefully they'll be happy to hear about all the fun you had. But either way, you know your loved one best, so temper the telling if you need to.

Of course you will need to discuss some particulars with your loved one, how to reach you in the case of an emergency, how they will be taking care of themselves while you're gone (whether that's someone else checking on them, or if they're self-reliant enough to do so on their own), and what responsibilities they'll need to handle while you're gone. Cell phones have made this all much easier, as texting and smartphones can make communication nearly seamless, but it's still a good idea to leave them alternate contact information just in case.

Finally, depending on their levels of self-reliance, your partner may need someone to check in while you're gone. Friends and loved ones are generally willing and able to take care of such check-ins, so don't be afraid to ask for help if you need it. You deserve the break, and your loved one will understand. Even if the fibro sufferer in your life doesn't need the help, letting local friends and loved ones know that you're going to be away can still be a good idea. It gives the fibro sufferer a backup if he or she becomes ill or needs help while you are away.

One recurring theme that fibro sufferers have is a need for reassurance. As mentioned earlier, the self-esteem and self-worth of many people with fibro takes a huge hit because they have lost so much that people, particularly Americans, use to define themselves. We are a working people, and when someone cannot work it's a huge hole that their self-worth dives into. Add to that the continual reminders that they look perfectly fine, and it's a recipe for disaster. I am honestly more surprised that there are people with fibro who *aren't* depressed than I am at the fact that the majority do get depressed.

How can you reassure the fibro sufferer in your life that they are worthy? Well, honestly, this will depend on them. For some, words of reassurance and love will be of primary importance. For others, gentle touches and contact will help them to maintain their confidence. Then there are those who find that actions speak louder than words, and they will be most reassured when you help them with chores or do things for them, like cooking or cleaning.

Often, communication is enhanced when you know what matters most to your person with fibro. If you want to know more about the way that you and your fibro sufferer communicate the best, there are articles online about the "Five Love Languages," and there is also a book by Gary Chapman called "The Five Love Languages" which can tell you and your loved one which type of communication you find the most emotionally impactful. This can help you to reassure them in the ways that matter most to them.

In general, though, if your fibro sufferer is feeling worthless or like they are a burden, the biggest thing you need to do is to understand that no matter how silly that seems to you, their feelings are valid and need to be acknowledged and respected. You can reassure them verbally, and also tell them the ways that they are valuable to you, but most often those of us with fibro just need to vent and feel heard. Of course, reassuring them that they do a lot more than they realize is also often helpful. Often, when I feel this way, my husband or a friend will list out the things I do for them and around the house, and I'm startled and pleased by the long litany of ways that I contribute. It is always good to be reminded that you matter, that you help, and that your contributions are noticed and valued.

Most often, though, the simplest way to reassure your loved one is to tell them that you love them. Sometimes, in the midst of depression, those three little words can mean the world.

Be compassionate, be loving, and know that your fibro sufferer values your help and care a great deal.

Chapter 19—Life goes on

One of the biggest things that grief counselors tell their patients is that getting back into a routine can help, because no matter how crushing the grief, life goes on. This is true for people with fibro, too. Establish a routine, learn your new limits, and find your way in your new life as quickly as you can. It will help you and those around you to adapt and make your way.

Keep in mind that no matter how difficult your life is now, it can and will get better. As you figure out your limitations and find the things that help you to mitigate your pain, you will be able to do more. And while you will never hit 'normal' again, you can still have a rich and fulfilling life.

Many people with fibro have had to quit "real" jobs, but there are ways to work that don't involve a nine-to-five job. I know crafters who sell their work on Etsy or Ebay, people who have gone into consulting so that they can work an unusual schedule, and people who changed careers because the only way they could work was to do something they truly loved.

Don't let fear of the pain stop you from living your life. You may have to adapt, but I know people with fibro who train horses, work construction, ice skate, lift weights, are stay at home moms, and who have chased their dreams in amazing ways. Find your passion, and let it guide you to the best life you can have.

Just as the saying goes, "living well is the best revenge," and living well with fibro is both possible and the best way to prevail over this illness.

For more information about fibro support groups, look around on Facebook, check your local hospital, or your nearby pain center to see if there's a fibro support group in your area.

About the Author

Kara Owl is a writer, sufferer with fibro, and a tarot reader with over 20 years of experience. She has written articles about living with fibro, about running a tarot business, and about healing with the tarot. She lives in Tallahassee, Florida with a husband, four cats, and a dog. Visit her website (owltakesflight.com) or Facebook page (www.facebook.com/WriterKaraOwl/) to learn more about her journey.

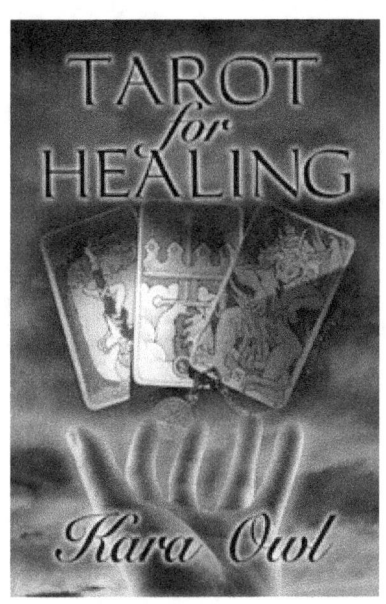

Tarot For Healing
by Kara Owl

Tarot for Healing will take you on a journey to health using the tarot. In these pages you'll find everything from first aid to in-depth healing using the magic of the Tarot Journey from the Fool all the way to the World.

Available in print and electronic format from all major book retailers.
Ebook $4.99/ Print $15.95

www.ingramcontent.com/pod-product-compliance
Lightning Source LLC
Chambersburg PA
CBHW072127280526
45788CB00002B/575